MOTHERKIND

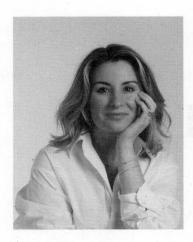

Zoe Blaskey is a mum of two, a qualified transformational coach, and the founder of Motherkind. Zoe is on a mission to help mothers shift from guilt, exhaustion, and comparison to confidence and calm – despite all the pressure and judgement of the modern world. She has coached thousands of mothers from overwhelmed to empowered using her Motherkind coaching methods.

Zoe hosts the critically acclaimed *Motherkind* podcast, which is one of the UK's top family podcasts with 5 million downloads and was named a 'top 10 podcast' by Apple. Every week Zoe interviews leading world experts such as Dr Becky, Glennon Doyle, Dr Gabor Maté, and Dr Rangan Chatterjee.

Zoe is a regular media contributor and has been featured in *Red*, *Stylist*, *The Times*, *Psychologies*, *SheerLuxe*, and the *Evening Standard*. *The Telegraph* celebrated the podcast as 'the antidote to the toxic perfectionism of modern motherhood'.

Zoe has two daughters and lives with her husband, Guy, by the sea in Dorset.

MOTHERKIND

Zoe Blaskey

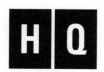

ONE PLACE. MANY STORIES

HQ
An imprint of HarperCollins*Publishers* Ltd
1 London Bridge Street
London SE1 9GF

www.harpercollins.co.uk

HarperCollins*Publishers*
Macken House, 39/40 Mayor Street Upper,
Dublin 1, D01 C9W8, Ireland

This edition 2024

2
First published in Great Britain by
HQ, an imprint of HarperCollins*Publishers* Ltd 2024

A catalogue record for this book is
available from the British Library.

HB ISBN: 978-0-00-865082-7

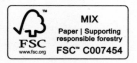

This book contains FSC˘ certified paper and other controlled
sources to ensure responsible forest management.

For more information visit: www.harpercollins.co.uk/green

This book is set in 11.7/16pt Minion by Type-it AS, Norway

Printed and Bound in the UK using 100% Renewable Electricity at
CPI Group (UK) Ltd, Croydon, CR0 4YY

For Guy, Jessie, and Rose
– my world

Contents

Welcome to *Motherkind*. This book aims to offer support on the various experiences linked to motherhood and women's health. While the book aims to offer help and guidance, this isn't a substitute for professional medical advice. We're all unique and individual experiences may vary so please always consult with your healthcare provider if you're worried about anything or are struggling. Our suggestions aren't endorsements, so feel free to do your own research before making any healthcare decisions. Let's journey through motherhood together with care and understanding.

Author's note

I have the privilege of including many of my coaching clients' stories in this book. Some have requested I change their names and details of their story; others have asked me to use their real names (in a desire to feel fully seen). All their stories are used with permission and much gratitude.

I have chosen to use the word 'mother' throughout this book, as that is how I identify. I use this term in the most inclusive way. I use child and children interchangeably, appreciating that some readers will have one child, others more.

Motherhood is not a monolith and, of course, this book doesn't speak for all mothers; that would be an impossible and futile task. Motherhood is shaped by your race, socioeconomic background, sexuality, relationship status, and every other intersection that exists. I speak to my own experience, my community's and clients' experiences, and the experts I have the privilege to include in this book. My greatest wish is that this book supports and helps you, but I know that I won't have captured everyone's lived experiences. Far from it. I am continually learning and unlearning how my own biases have impacted me, and I hope that I continue to do so for as long as I do this work.

How to use this book

This isn't a book about how to do things my way; I've read enough of those to know their limitations. This is a book about empowering *you*. The more I learn, the more I understand that there are very few universal answers, and I would never proclaim to know what is right for you. But I can help you find some of those answers for yourself, by sharing the things I've learned along the way.

Each chapter includes three ways to support yourself:

- Motherkind Moments: concepts or ideas explained in bitesize ways.
- Motherkind Musings: self-coaching questions that will unlock your self-awareness and insight.
- Motherkind Toolkits: coaching tools that will help you implement the concepts or ideas into your own life.

I would really encourage you to grab a notebook and jot down your thoughts to the Motherkind musing questions as you go through the book. Writing down your thoughts and feelings is magical because it takes the swirling thoughts from your mind and puts them somewhere visible: the page. It's the best way I know to uncover new insights, self-awareness, and clarity – it takes hardly any time and it's free. If you've never done this before, do expect to feel some resistance, but do it anyway. If you're worried about it being read, you can throw it away. It's the process of writing that has value, not keeping it. My clients tell me they can't believe the breakthroughs they've had by simply writing down their thoughts, and each of the Musing questions has been crafted and tested (many times) to help you get the most insight in the quickest time.

At the end of each chapter is a five-minute summary, for those days when you need help but haven't got time to read the whole section. These summaries are great to return to time and time again, because if you're anything like me when I get busy, I forget what I've read.

One last thing, because I've read so many of these types of books and I've thought, wow, that author must have the best life, a life with no challenges or struggles. I've used books like these to beat myself up more. I want you to know that even though I'm known as a motherhood 'expert', I still struggle every single day. Every day a new challenge comes up for me, such is the nature of mothering, and I flounder, often. I'm learning right alongside you and trust me when I say that I've written the book I need myself. There is no one book or expert out there that will solve all your problems or give you a dream life. Please don't put me or this book on that pedestal, because we will have a very long way to fall. Think of this book as a buffet: there'll be bits you love, bits you hate, bits you want to try again, and bits you want to learn to cook at home. Take what you like and leave the rest on the table.

Introduction: We need a new way

'You will always feel the most lost right before you find your way again.'

ANON

I'm sitting on the floor in my living room, my eleven-month-old daughter is red-faced and crying, and I'm trying my best to calm her. I'm doing all the things I've been told to do – hugging her, singing to her, trying to work out what could be upsetting her – but it's not making any difference. I feel utterly alone, panicked by this beautiful ball of emotion in front of me. I can feel a tightness coming over my chest, my nervous system is flooded, and I want to run away. Except I don't really want to run away. I want to be present, grounded, and calm so I can help my beautiful daughter. Suddenly I remember to breathe. I take some deep breaths, I feel my system settle, and unsurprisingly she settles too.

Calmer now, I sit there thinking about how broken I feel. Both physically from way too little sleep for way too long, and emotionally from feeling lost. I feel defeated from trying to mother 'perfectly'. I'm continually getting stuck in cycles of guilt and wondering just how damaged my daughter is going to be from having a broken mother like me. My world feels like it's been turned upside down and inside out, but no one else seems to be struggling. I don't even know who I am anymore. So, I fall back on one of my oldest coping strategies:

making everything look good on the outside while trying to ignore the mess I feel inside.

My inner critic was raging, my confidence was at its lowest ebb in a decade, and no part of me felt worthy to raise the beautiful soul I had in my arms. The love I felt for her was showing me the lack of love I felt for myself. It was like motherhood was a magnifying glass for my broken parts.

I looked around at the many parenting books scattered across the messy kitchen. My tired eyes scanned them, looking for comforting words to explain how I was feeling, but all I found was more pressure, more rules and more reasons to feel guilty and overwhelmed. I thought that there was something wrong with me.

None of the books gave me the words of comfort and reassurance I really needed. They didn't explain how to stop feeling so guilty, or why I was obsessing over every tiny decision, or how to quieten my inner critic.

A quick Google search confirmed my fears. I was told I needed to 'bounce back' and 'drink more gin'. If words make worlds, then where were the kind, compassionate words that felt fitting for this new world I found myself in? Loving my child was the easy part, it was everything else I found hard. The guilt, the perfectionism, the fear, the control, the constant inner critic, the never-ending advice, the mental load, the work/life juggle, and how every relationship in my life had changed. But no one seemed to be talking about it.

So, I decided that I would.

Fuelled by passion, confusion, and a selfish need to feel the promised joy in motherhood, I started a podcast. I bought a cheap microphone and begged some of the wisest minds across the world to speak to me. I called it *Motherkind*, because what I needed most was my own kindness, and to stop telling myself that there was something wrong with me. The podcast, which started in nap times, has now been listened to over five million times. *Motherkind* has been a word-of-mouth success spread through WhatsApp groups, GP surgeries, toddler classes, and social media, and has so far reached 150 countries.

I've spoken to the world's best across many disciplines, including parenting, psychology, sociology, anthropology, neuroscience and philosophy. I've interviewed experts from all over the world, spoken to thousands of mothers about their experiences, and coached hundreds more.

There is nothing new about my struggles, but this is part of the problem. I now know that it is almost universally whispered, sometimes just to ourselves, that motherhood is hard. And I understand why it's a whisper, not a shout: because children are a gift. So many women who want children devastatingly struggle to conceive. So, we keep quiet about the hard parts, almost out of respect and reverence. But we do need to talk about it. We need to talk about how we can support ourselves through this incredible journey, and we can't expect to know how to navigate one of the biggest transitions in our lives without the right tools.

Understanding how to ride the emotional rollercoaster of motherhood changed everything for me. I found my confidence, turned my inner critic into an inner coach, learned how to manage my stress and energy, and found more joy and freedom in motherhood than I ever dreamed possible. I started becoming the type of woman and mother I wanted to be and who I want my children to see.

You hold in your hands the knowledge I've learned – tried, tested, and proven to support mothers. And this is what I know to be true: there was nothing wrong with me; I was finding it hard because it *is* hard. I was finding it hard because no one had taught me how to challenge the expectations of motherhood, to do it my way. I've coached thousands of women who've gone from feeling totally broken by motherhood to feeling empowered, confident, and clearer about themselves and their lives than ever before. I am lucky enough to get messages every day from mothers telling me how the ideas I share have transformed their lives. Most of the ideas aren't mine – I stand on the shoulders of giants. I've learned from the best in the world, and used my coaching expertise to create simple tools that can change your day, week, or even your life.

I've created exactly the resource I wished I'd had when I was sitting on my living room floor that day. I've condensed thousands of hours spent researching, reading, training, and interviewing into simple, applicable, time-efficient tools that you can start using straight away to feel more present, happy, and clear – despite the insane pressure of life as a mother in today's world.

If you've picked up this book, or maybe a friend has passed it to you, you're likely to be feeling tested by motherhood. Maybe you feel like you've lost a sense of who you are or what matters to you. Maybe you feel resentful towards your partner or co-parent because you feel like it's always you who is picking up the pieces and keeping the ship afloat. Maybe motherhood has brought-up challenges from your own childhood, and you have no idea what to do about it. Maybe you are exhausted because you feel too guilty to say no. Maybe you feel overwhelmed at the sheer relentlessness of it all. Or maybe you just want some reassurance, validation, and new ideas. The pages you hold in your hands will support, guide, and help you with all of this and much more.

It doesn't matter how old your children are. This book has tools that will help mothers of ten-day-olds and ten-year-olds. Because the premise of this book is not what's going on with your children, but what's going on with you.

This isn't a parenting book. I'm not going to tell you how to wean your toddler, or why your six-year-old won't sleep, or how to manage screen time. Because I'm not a parenting expert. I'm an expert in helping you: the mother.

My sole focus is on you. Take a deep breath and let that sink in. I bet you've read loads of books about how to help your children, but in order to be the most effective, loving, present mother you want to be, you have to focus on yourself, too.

I believe motherhood is one of the most important and yet under-supported roles in the world. I want that to change. Our societies, institutions, and governments do not support mothers in the way they need to, and this needs to change. But systemic change takes decades, and you need help now. So, this book is going to focus on what's in your control, right now, in this moment.

We need a different way. A different way to support mothers, and a different way to support ourselves.

Many of us have been handed down the selfless mother map, the one that tells us the only thing that matters is our child and that we need to be constantly working inside or outside the home to have value. The one that instils the belief that motherhood is natural and easy, and any feelings that differ are wrong and shameful and need to be quickly swept under the crumb-stained carpet. I got the memo that to be a good mother I had to do it all, be it all, and love it all without complaining or explaining. It told me that while I should wish for my children to be happy, I shouldn't care about my own happiness because, as the mother, I didn't matter.

But every time I ignored my needs, didn't make space for my feelings, and chose the comfort of others over advocating for myself, I took a wrong turn. And it left me broken. This new map is going to show you how to ignore the signs pointing towards martyrdom, perfectionism, people pleasing, guilt, and control. Instead, it will show you new paths pointing towards self-worth, confidence, self-value, and protecting your time and energy. Following these paths will guide you towards a life filled with more energy, more confidence, and more joy.

What we need, our children need, and ultimately the world needs, is empowered mothers.

To follow this new map, we need to understand the terrain – the lay of the land. Knowing that we're standing on uneven ground will help us to forgive ourselves when we wobble. Understanding the landscape we're mothering in will give us self-compassion.

We're the first generation of mothers raising our children with social media while grappling with a post-pandemic world during a young person's mental health crisis. We've lost our village, we're facing crippling childcare costs, and we're often mothering without support from our families. More of us are working more than ever before, yet we're still taking on the majority of the emotional and invisible labour at home. We're more connected digitally, yet lonelier than ever. We know more than ever before about the profound importance of the first five years of a child's life, but we don't have the support systems in place to implement this knowledge, so we feel like we're failing constantly. The explosion of the parenting industry has meant that we think we should instantly be able to pull out the 'perfect' script, word, or soothing tone – despite how we might be feeling within ourselves.

This book is going to show you – in spite of this rugged, stormy terrain – how to feel better, happier, more joyful, and connected to yourself and others by focusing on what you can control. It's going to show you how to use boundaries to get your time and energy back. It's going to teach you how to finally quieten that voice in your head that says you're not doing it right or you can't cope. It's going to show you how to free yourself from guilt and be able to focus on what's really important to you and your family.

My deepest hope is that this book will be a thousand invitations, springing up from every page, calling you to leave behind the heavy weight of guilt, pressure, and exhaustion, and instead recraft a motherhood steeped in self-belief, trust, and worth. In case no one has told you already today: you are incredible. You're performing the most important and yet undervalued role in the world. I see you, and I think you're a wonder. Now let's get you believing that as well.

We are stronger together. To join the movement, go to Motherkind.co for additional resources and downloads, and use the hashtag #motherkind when sharing this book and the ideas within it so I can thank you and follow your journey.

Chapter One: Motherhood is meant to change you

'Becoming a mother leaves no woman as it found her. It unravels her and rebuilds her. It cracks her open, takes her to her edges. It's both beautiful and brutal, often at the same time.'

NIKKI MCCAHON, MATRESCENCE EDUCATOR

I don't know who first said 'words create worlds', but they were right. When we can't find the right words to fit our experience it leaves us feeling lost and alone. We grab for words that might not quite feel right, and just like trying to squeeze ourselves into a too-small shoe, it's uncomfortable and we know it isn't right. But at least it's something. This was my experience. I couldn't find the right words to put to my experience of becoming a mother, so I did what I'd been trained as a woman to do – ignore it and smile on through. I have observed, almost universally, that when women don't have the words or understanding for an experience, we blame ourselves. We decide there must be something wrong with us.

I close the door behind me and feel the cold air against my hot skin. It feels odd not to be wrangling the buggy out the door, mentally checking through my kit list (nappies, wipes, nappy bags, dummies, spare clothes, muslins, bottle, spare bottle...) as I try not to think about how bone tired I am. Instead of the changing bag I've flung only a small handbag over my shoulder, and it feels like a third heavy limb is missing. It's my first coffee with a friend since becoming a mother – a completely normal Saturday-morning activity pre-motherhood. But walking down the road, nothing feels the same. My body is different, my relationship is different, my priorities are completely different, and I'm not with the new love of my life. But my mind is consumed with thoughts of her. Is she okay? Will I get back in time to pump? Will Guy, my husband, be okay looking after her? Am I enjoying this? Should I be enjoying this more? Why does everything seem louder? Why do I feel so angry? Am I anxious? I'm walking along the same road, wearing the same shoes, and heading to the same coffee shop, but nothing feels the same. It was then that it hit me, like a lightning bolt of clarity: I will never be the same again. I won't ever get back to the 'old' me. How can I? I have grown, birthed, and am responsible for another human. I am changed.

I loved being pregnant. It was one of those annoyingly easy, non-complicated pregnancies and births. My challenges came once my little girl was in my arms. Even after the hormonal dust settled, I didn't feel right. I felt like a stranger to myself. I felt like I didn't 'fit' my new role. I felt awkward pushing the buggy down the road. I didn't know how to be me anymore. My clothes didn't fit. My daily routine was unrecognisable from the buzzing, busy days of working in the city. I found those early newborn days overwhelmingly boring and intense. I have never been more busy and more bored in my life. I adored my little girl, almost to the point of obsession. It was the changes happening within me that felt like I was putting on a suit that didn't belong to me. I remember when I was a little girl putting on my mum's high heels and necklaces, pretending to be grown up – that's how I felt as a new mother. Like I was performing a role, one I didn't think I was very good at it. I struggled with breastfeeding, and my inner critic had a field day about it. 'See,' I heard it say. 'I knew you couldn't do this.' Did I have postnatal depression, I wondered? But what I did know for sure was that I felt different.

No one else seemed to be talking about this feeling of irreversible change. So, I pushed it down. Far down. I smiled and went to baby groups. I pushed down the anger I felt towards my husband as he slept soundly next to me while I grappled in the dark at 3 a.m. trying to get the latch right. I pushed down the feelings of confusion, of disorientation, of a growing chasm of who I was before and who stared back at me in the mirror with a baby on her hip. I felt such shame at my cocktail of feelings – deep joy for this incredible baby in my arms, but also anger, fear, anxiety, and confusion bubbling just under the surface. I had no idea then, but I know now that what I was experiencing was completely normal and that almost every mother will experience the same emotional marbling in early motherhood.

The problem is when we keep quiet about it. We deny it even to ourselves by painting on a smile instead of having the courage to let the mask drop even for a moment. I wish I'd known then that it's normal to feel completely joyful and completely disoriented at exactly the same time.

Motherkind Moment
It's completely normal to feel overwhelmingly joyful and utterly disoriented at the same time.

Before motherhood I would dart around, from work meetings to meeting friends, relatively stress free. Yet in those early months my life became very small, and I barely left my local area. I remember when my eldest daughter was five months old I really wanted to go to a particular yoga workshop, but it was right across the other side of my city. It took me weeks to build up to it, planning my every move and eventuality. It struck me, as I was setting out on what felt like a brave quest with my baby in a sling, how I would have done this journey before motherhood without even giving it a thought. I am changed. My controlling, perfectionist side that I had worked so hard in a decade of therapy to shift came back stronger than ever, like an unwelcome sequel. The mood music of my early days of motherhood was that I didn't feel good enough – not good enough for my daughter, perhaps not even cut out for motherhood. I now know that I'm not alone, having spoken to many doctors, psychologists, and parenting experts who have told me they felt exactly the same in the early months and years. Dr Zoe Williams, general practitioner and author, told me on the podcast, 'I thought I'd be prepared, but so many times I thought: I just can't do this. I had a lot of self-doubt and anxiety. It really surprised me how hard I found it.' And Jessica VanderWier, child therapist, told me, 'I had eight years of post-secondary education in mental health, and I was still blown away by how anxious I felt and how unprepared I really felt for motherhood.'

Fast forward a year and I started the *Motherkind* podcast in a desperate quest to understand motherhood and myself better. I booked a guest called Dr Oscar Serrallach, an Australian doctor who was making waves with his work on the postnatal period. I messed up booking a venue to record the episode, so we ended up recording in my car on a boiling-hot day and we couldn't have the air conditioning on because of the noise. I was obviously mortified by my lack of organization and unprofessionalism. There we were, sweating and talking, when he said a word that would completely change my view of myself and motherhood: *matrescence*, or as I like to think of it, the word that changed my life.

We've all heard of adolescence, right? Of course we have, we've all been through it. I remember it as a time of much soul searching and identity shifting (anyone else try on a few different identities before feeling at home in your own self? I vividly remember pretending to like Smashing Pumpkins in an effort to fit in with the grunge crew at school. I'd listen to Kylie the moment I got home). We typically support our teens going through this shift, or at least try to. We know it's a bumpy time, when friendships change, relationships change – everything changes. It's a time when we're no longer a child, but not yet an adult – it's the gap between the two. And the question we constantly ask ourselves during this time is, 'Who am I?' Adolescence is a time when, if well supported, you emerge more... you. Well, matrescence is exactly the same process but it describes becoming a mother. Only added to the dictionary in 2019, Cambridge Dictionary describes it as: 'The process of becoming a mother.' When I first heard the word delivered in a gorgeous, kind Australian accent that Saturday morning in a sweaty car, my shoulders dropped and my shame instantly lessened. I was filled with self-compassion. The messy, complicated cocktail of feelings I had, were all encapsulated in one word: matrescence.

Motherkind Moment

Matrescence describes the developmental process of becoming a mother. It's a time of change on almost every level: physical, hormonal, economic, social, emotional, and spiritual.

Turns out I wasn't doing it wrong at all; I was going through my matrescence. This phase was meant to be a messy, bumpy transition, and a time of questioning, identity crises, and confusion, plus a cocktail of emotions and hormonal shifts. When I asked the Motherkind community about the impact of hearing this word on the podcast, I received hundreds of messages. The common theme was: 'I no longer feel like I'm failing, that I "should" have done better, knowing this word has replaced self-criticism with self-compassion.'

Why had I never heard of this word before? Despite it being coined in 1973 by anthropologist Dana Raphael, it had never made it to the mainstream and was instead hidden in medical textbooks and academic circles. I'd read all the books, signed up for an antenatal course, even done pregnancy yoga teacher training, but not one person had ever mentioned this word or process. Even as I am writing this, the wriggly red lines are ever present under the word – 'Unrecognized word,' my laptop tells me confidently. Oh, the irony.

Everyone's matrescence is different, but every woman entering into motherhood has one. However you arrive at motherhood – adoption, surrogacy, fertility treatment, step parenting, and every other way it's possible to become a mother – you go through matrescence. And we can have a different matrescence experience with each child. Lotte Jeffs, author of *The Queer Parent*, told me, 'It took me five years to feel light again after my wife gave birth to our daughter.'

You might have found your matrescence easy. You might have found it completely discombobulating, like I did. But in a society that doesn't understand or support our transition to motherhood, it's vital we do this for ourselves. Matrescence is a process and there's conflicting views from the experts on how long it lasts. Some say up to ten years, while others think it lasts forever. So if you're reading this, it's likely you will be in or about to enter your matrescence. And if you have a male partner, then they too will be in their patrescence, which is the transition into fatherhood.

When I discovered matrescence, I realized that being a mother was not just about my child and how I showed up for her, but also about me and how I showed up for myself in this new season of my life. Lucy Jones, author of *Matrescence*, told me: 'It was the most physical but also psychological, emotional, spiritual, existential, socio-political experience of my whole life. And it blew away everything I thought I knew about myself, about the world, about the things I've been taught.'

I'm so passionate about this word because there are so many mothers who think there's something wrong with them for feeling the very normal confusion and identity shifts that motherhood brings. When we become mothers it's as if everything in our lives gets thrown up in the air – our identities, our relationships, our time, our bodies, our sense of what's important, our goals, our dreams. Matrescence is the process we go through to put all that back together again in a new way, piece by piece like a jigsaw puzzle, only with no image on the box to copy. Amy Taylor-Kabbaz, author of *Mama Rising*, told me on the podcast, 'It's this period of time where you are undoing who you were, and becoming who you are going to become, but you aren't there yet.' We need to stop expecting mothers to glide and slide easily into motherhood, all joy and florals – it's just not that way at all. Motherhood is the one thing in your life that changes everything around you.

Motherkind Community: Clare's story

'I wasn't crazy after all; I was living through a massive transition. And my goodness did I feel angry! Of course I was stressed out and a mess – society had not supported me, and I had been denied important truths. Motherhood can be a beautiful, rewarding, and fulfilling experience, while at the same time being difficult, messy, scary, and very tiring. How had I never heard any of this before?'

Recently while on holiday I had a moment of madness (or was it my looming fortieth birthday?) and decided on a whim to tick off a bucket list experience: paragliding. I'd always wondered what it would feel like to be a thousand feet up in the air with nothing more than a kite between me and the end of it all. I am also determined to show my two young girls that midlife motherhood does not mean the end of new adventures and of trying things for the first time. So, I booked it and off I went. I jumped excitedly into the minibus, embarrassed yet again at my lack of language skills as I tried to get by in my broken Spanish with the other paragliders.

I felt calm and excited as we headed off up the winding road towards the mountain I would shortly be launching myself off. Suddenly we pulled into a disused car park, no mention of why or what we'd be doing there. The driver jumped out, leaving us tourists looking at each other with that turned-down mouth and slight shake of the head that says, 'I have no idea either.' I felt my heart start to beat a little faster. How long would we be here? Why had we stopped? It was the uncertainty, the not knowing that got my palms sweaty and my mind racing. After about ten minutes the driver got back in and without saying a word, we carried on up the hill. We arrived at the top and without any briefing or direction, everyone left the van. I followed. I assumed we'd all sit around with some clip boards and instructions before we jumped off into the sky, but no. We were given a few simple instructions and a harness to put on and before I knew it, I was running towards the edge of a mountain with an instructor strapped behind me. I will never forget that first moment after jumping off; time stood still as we floated up into the clouds. But I couldn't stop thinking about landing – I hadn't been told where or how this would happen. Not knowing what was going to happen was ruining the experience.

The one thing our brains hate more than anything is uncertainty. Lowering down towards the landing point, I was told to 'just run when we hit the ground'. As we glided in towards the black sand, all I could hear was my heartbeat reverberating around my head. We landed easily and I immediately thought, that would have been so much more incredible if I'd known what was going to happen. And so it is with matrescence; it would have been so much more incredible if I'd known what was going to happen.

In motherhood we are thrown all the clichés like unwelcome

confetti as we walk down the street with a bump, baby, or toddler. 'Enjoy every minute.' 'You've got your hands full!' 'Sleep when the baby sleeps.' These throwaway words are not only unhelpful, but they also gloss over the lived experience of the majority of mothers. A survey of 3,600 women by the app Peanut revealed that 75 per cent of respondents felt invisible once they became mothers.[1] Of course they do – we are completely unprepared for the reality of what motherhood really entails. Imagine if you knew *before* motherhood that you were going to go through your matrescence – that it was going to be messy, and complicated, and you would feel changed but that was to be expected, and that there was nothing wrong with you – it was *your* process. As reproductive psychiatrist and author of *What No One Tells You* Dr Alexandra Sacks says, 'Too many women are ashamed to speak openly about their complicated experiences for fear of being judged. This type of social isolation may even trigger postpartum depression.'

Imagine if people asked you 'How is your matrescence going?' 'How are you navigating the massive transition?' 'Do you have enough support?' Imagine if we held the hands of women and told them of the shift that was coming their way and gave them tools, ideas, validation, and support to navigate it. Can you imagine if teens were expected to go through adolescence alone? Worse still, can you imagine if we didn't tell teens about adolescence and left them to navigate these huge changes with no prior understanding or support. But this is what women in developed countries are expected to do. Amy Taylor-Kabbaz told me on the podcast that in many other cultures there were 'ancient ways that women used to welcome new mothers into this process. We used to sit together in a circle and be passed down this wisdom'. It's a myth that mothers should just 'know' how to care for our children. As Chelsea Conaboy, author of *Mother Brain,* told me, 'We are led to believe as mothers there is an unused part of our brain that suddenly gets turned on when we become mothers and that's called "instinct", which will mean that we know what to do, that mothering is easy and natural and innate. That is a *myth*. We learn how to mother and how to live our lives as mothers – through knowledge and experience.'

Can you imagine if we got this word and all it encapsulates into the mainstream? How empowering it would be for mothers and everyone that cares for us? Could we be the generation of mothers who will refuse to let the women following behind us not understand this vital process and empower them to get the support they need? I think we can.

Internationally renowned speaker and author on trauma, health, and human development Dr Gabor Maté told me on the podcast that it isn't what we experience that determines its impact on us, it's how *supported we feel* with what we experience. This matters.

Motherkind Moment

We could be the generation of mothers to help matrescence become mainstream.

Motherkind Musing

We only gain wisdom and insight through processing our experiences. Tempting as it is to skip this, I encourage you to spend a couple of moments thinking about the following questions:

If you're already a mother:
- How is your matrescence going?
- What have you learned about yourself?
- What words of support and kindness do you need to hear from yourself about your transition to motherhood?

If you're pregnant or soon to become a mother:
- How has learning about matrescence helped you?
- What support do you think you will need?
- What words of support and kindness do you need to hear from yourself about your transition to motherhood?

'I just feel so sad,' my client said to me. 'I struggled so much in those early years. I wasn't myself. I hated my partner and, at times, I hated myself.' I introduced her to the idea of matrescence and told her that the process of becoming a mother is a messy, complicated cocktail of conflicting emotions and fears. I could see the tears already forming in her eyes. We all need recognition, and it's an honour to give my coaching clients this. When we recognize a truth that we've pushed down, the relief often comes in tears. 'I thought I was a bad person, a bad mother,' she said. I'm crying as I write these words to you now, because of how heartbreaking it is that so many mothers feel like this – like failures. We're left alone to figure out the greatest transition a woman can go through, and left to our own devices, we decide we're failures. I suggested she write a letter to herself, forgiving herself for the self-criticism. 'I want to write knowing what I now know, telling myself then that she was okay after all. She wasn't a bad mother for feeling so many complex emotions.' My client has said she now looks back on that time completely differently – with compassionate, kind eyes. When we first started working together, she wasn't sure she wanted another baby because she felt she got it so 'wrong' the first time. She's now pregnant with her second child. Words matter.

Motherkind Toolkit: Compassionate letter writing

Compassionate letter writing to yourself is a powerful coaching tool I will suggest a few times in this book, because my clients tell me how transformational this simple exercise has been for them. It might feel odd if you've never done it before, but if you can keep writing for a couple of minutes, you will find your flow and gain a deeper insight into your emotions. You don't need to keep it if you're worried about confidentiality – it's the process of writing it that provides the benefits.

If you're already a mother: Write a letter to your new-mother self, forgiving her for what she didn't know, releasing any self-blame, criticism, or judgement with the kindest, most compassionate words you can find.

If you're pregnant or soon to become a mother: Write a letter to your future new-mother self; tell her how you will support and care for her through her matrescence.

Motherkind Community: Arianna's story

'My matrescence started during pregnancy. I suffered antenatal depression in the early weeks and went from being fiercely independent and level-headed to needy and volatile. I couldn't recognize myself or my behaviour, and I suffered a less-than-ideal birthing experience, the aftermath of which dragged into the first few months of motherhood. My brain wasn't right, I didn't feel good, and once my son was born everyone kept asking me if I "loved it", and all I kept thinking was, "No, I don't. I love him, but I don't love motherhood." Nothing came naturally to me, and I found everything really hard. I wanted quick fixes and control, neither of which existed with a newborn. I was scared of so much: his cries, being alone with him, going into bedtime, getting it wrong or messing him up. I was even scared of the fabric baby sling! I tried to get it on once, but it didn't work, and I cried for an entire afternoon. I laugh now, but I felt like a failure in almost everything I did.'

As well as feeling scared, Arianna also remembered feeling angry:

'I was angry that my son cried so much, angry that I couldn't soothe him any other way than using my boobs, angry at my wonderful co-parenting partner who took extended paternity leave but robbed me of a "normal" maternity experience. I held onto so much resentment towards him for finding parenting easier than me, for not being so triggered by our son's cries, for keeping calm when I couldn't.'

Arianna found herself catastrophizing every moment, and one negative thought would spiral out of control and lead to more harmful thoughts that left her feeling anxious, ashamed, guilty, and worthless. The most pivotal thing Arianna learned about her own matrescence was understanding the importance of awareness. She learned to notice her thoughts and reactions, and that gave her the space to question them.

'That was step one to helping me feel differently. Once I was aware of how I was reacting to something, I could change my reaction to it. Then once I was aware of something, I learned to approach it through the lens of compassion rather than critique so that I could speak back to myself in a kinder and more forgiving way. I learned how to reframe situations and see them for what they are rather than what my mind perceived them to be. I developed the patience to take a deep breath and decide how I wanted to react to something, and in doing so started to regulate my emotions. I've come to realize that parenting is not about raising my son at all; it's about re-raising myself. There's nothing I need to "fix" in him. Instead, I need to repair and rewire my old thought patterns and behaviours. This understanding has changed my entire energy towards my son, myself, and motherhood.'

Stop looking backwards, you're not going that way

It would probably win me more friends at the nursery and school gates to nod along with the 'you'll get your old self back' trope, but I don't buy into that at all. I want you to think about any major transition, any challenge, any heart-expanding experience you've been through – it changes you. It has to. When you become a mother, you also become a new version of yourself.

So, I'm going to ask you to think about this differently – you don't get your 'old' self back. You're changed. You've been through so much already in motherhood and it has shown you qualities in yourself that maybe you would never have developed otherwise. I've listened to thousands of mothers' stories, and I know one thing for sure: every single one of those mothers found a strength they didn't know they had through a challenge they didn't know they'd face. Maybe it's the courage to keep trying for a baby after three miscarriages (if that isn't real courage then I don't know what is, and sadly I know from personal experience). Maybe it's the surrender and trust you learned after your birth was completely different to how you expected it to be. Maybe it's the soul-stirring intimacy you've experienced for the first time while looking into the eyes of your child. Maybe it's the strength you've found to protect your child from harm. Maybe it's the vulnerability you've found to ask for help for the first time in your adult life. Maybe it's the strength you found to keep opening your heart to your baby in ICU, never knowing from one day to the next whether your open heart would ever mend should the unimaginable happen. Maybe it's the hope you found after round after round of failed fertility treatment. Maybe you've found your voice and found yourself roaring 'no' when someone has tried to cross the line with your child. Maybe it's the first time you've ever really considered loving yourself, seeing the depth of love mirrored back at you in your toddler's eyes (how can you be so loved and not have it pierce the veil of your harshness with yourself?).

Every mother I know has struggled in matrescence, whether it was with fertility, birth, feeding, relationships, or postpartum. No, you won't get your 'old' self back – you've been through too much to do that disservice to yourself. I won't let you. Your old self is a shadow of the woman you've become and are becoming. It's time to honour that. I refuse to buy into the narrative that we go through this life-giving, expansive, transformative experience of motherhood and listen to the offensive narrative from the world that we have to 'get back' to our old selves.

Your baby lives on in you

I sadly had two miscarriages between the births of my first and second daughters and both were traumatic experiences. I wish I'd known about feto-maternal chimerism, when the foetus sends stem cells into the mother. Researchers believe that these stem cells can heal parts of the mother's body that are damaged, which is truly beautiful. Even more striking is that long after the baby is born, these foetal cells continue to have a positive effect on the mother's body. The cells, full of our children's DNA, collect in our hearts, our brains, and everywhere we can think of.[2] They become part of us, often staying with us for decades. This is true even if the baby we carried didn't live to be born. I take so much comfort from knowing that the cells of my four babies may live on in me.

Motherkind Musing

- What qualities have you developed in motherhood?
- How have the challenges you've faced helped you to develop these qualities?

Your brain changes, too

There have been some recent discoveries that prove what us mothers have known for millennia – our brains are changed forever by motherhood. Our brains change more in pregnancy and postpartum than at any other time in our lives, including adolescence. In fact, they change so dramatically that in one study, a computer could detect who had been pregnant based on brain scans alone.[3] Chelsea Conaboy, author of *Mother Brain*, told me, 'We are remade by parenthood. Becoming a parent changes our brain functionally and structurally in ways that shape our physical and mental health over the *remainder of our life.*'

Our brains change to make us more protective, empathetic, and emotionally attuned.[4,5] This idea is far from the 'baby brain' trope with its negative connotations of forgetfulness, and there is growing evidence that motherhood is actually good for our brains, or 'neuroprotective'. Conaboy told me on the podcast, 'It actually makes sense that parenthood could be beneficial for our brains. Raising children requires us to constantly deal with new challenges, to change and change again. Couldn't it be that this is a kind of cognitive enrichment? Research, in humans and in other animals, suggests that it is.'

You're not meant to 'bounce back' – you are not a ball

A while ago I saw a video on social media of Victoria Beckham being weighed live on television to see if she had lost her baby weight at just eight weeks postpartum. This was filmed only twenty-three years ago. Many in our generation of mothers would have watched it. It would never happen now, hopefully, but it's so important to remember that this pressure to 'bounce back' is in our psyche. And it's our subconscious mind that influences our beliefs and behaviour, not what we consciously think.

Nothing enrages me more than the idea of us 'bouncing back'. It started with the idea of celebrities bouncing back from a physical perspective, but now permeates so many areas of motherhood. Bounce back has come to mean getting back to your pre-motherhood self as quickly as possible. The accepted 'wisdom' is that as soon as you have a baby the gun fires on the race to get back to who you were before as quickly as possible, both physically and mentally. It's celebrated everywhere from headlines to baby groups. The dictionary definition of bounce back is to 'recover quickly from a setback'. The language we use matters; our children are not a 'setback'. The very notion that we are supposed to go through the greatest transition imaginable and then bounce back as if it never happened – to fit back into our lives, our jeans, and our old identities – is, I believe, why so many of us feel we are getting it wrong and why we blame ourselves.

Why does it fire me up so much? Because it's a visceral example of how motherhood has come to be so devalued in our modern Western world. We're told we have to be exactly the same person we were before, just with a baby perched on our hip, and yet again women are reduced to what we look like. We're performing the incredible feats of birthing, raising, moulding, and loving the next generation, but what seems to matter is how quickly we can get our pre-baby jeans back on. Just think for a moment how absurd this is. We're so indoctrinated with this rubbish; we even start to buy into it ourselves. I'm not talking about exercise here – I'm not actually talking about physical appearance at all. I'm talking about the very idea that has been so insidiously planted into the narrative of motherhood that the ultimate goal is to get back to where we were before as quickly as possible – to work, into our jeans, into our old routines. I call bullshit. Amy Taylor-Kabbaz, author of *Mama Rising*, told me, 'When the culture and society around her hasn't allowed her to see herself as changing, has actually asked her not to change … it's like trying to hold a teenager down as a child, like treating them like a child when they're changing before your eyes.'

This matters, because studies have found that women who experienced pressure to 'bounce back' after giving birth reported poorer mental health.[6] So, if our brains are changed and we can't revert to who we were before, shouldn't we focus on moving forward?

A new way to think about identity

Many mothers have said to me over the years, 'I just don't know who I am anymore.' I think most are surprised by my answer: that a crisis of identity is part of matrescence, and actually a completely normal part of motherhood. Any major life change can trigger an identity crisis – redundancy, career change, divorce, marriage, relocation – and societally there is an acceptance and understanding of that. Our identities are never 'set' because we are always changing. I have identified as a schoolgirl, economics undergraduate, single woman, party girl – none of which are true now. The identities we wear transform and are replaced as we grow through life, just like our children outgrowing their clothes. Allowing yourself to gently explore what it means to you to add 'mother' to your identity is a gift to yourself. But because of the bounce-back culture we operate in, we can wrongly assume there is something wrong with us when we find ourselves thinking, 'Who even am I?' I want to shout this from the rooftops: there is *nothing* wrong with you or your identity crisis. Your values and identity are *supposed* to change in motherhood. Author and podcaster Millie Mackintosh told me, 'I am unrecognisable from my pre-motherhood self.'

When we don't know who we are anymore, we long to return to the familiar; our old identities can feel like a life raft on the wild waves of motherhood. With 94 per cent of mothers saying they feel their identity has been reduced to just one – mother[7] – it's clear we need a new way to approach identity in motherhood. Instead of grappling with the question 'Who am I?' I think we need a better one: 'I wonder who I'm becoming now?'

When we lead with curiosity, we open ourselves up to a gentler way of exploring ourselves. All change involves a loss, and in the case of matrescence, it's the loss of a former version of ourselves. All loss involves grief, so it's entirely expected that we might grieve the loss of our former selves. Grieving the loss of carefree, responsibility-free days doesn't make you an ungrateful mother any more than grieving the loss of childhood makes you an ungrateful adult. It's all part of the process.

Motherkind Moment

It is completely normal to struggle with identity changes in motherhood.

Donna Lancaster, therapist and author of *Wise Words for Women*, told me, 'You can't get to the new without letting go of the old and I think that's true when we become mothers. There's a grieving process of the life that we had before we became a mother, no matter how much we might have wanted to become a mother. There's a grieving process that that identity is over. She's gone; the woman you were before you became a mother has gone. And she will not return. So many women feel shame because they say, "But I'm so lucky that I've got this perfect baby." It's not either/or. It's both. You can be incredibly grateful and feel incredibly blessed that you are to have the miracle of a child (especially when so many women aren't able to conceive who want to). But it doesn't mean you're not also able to say, "*and* I miss the freedom of being just myself, not a mother first and foremost."'

It might seem self-indulgent to feel side swept at your loss of
identity and the need to grieve the loss of your former self, but it's far
from it. It's actually vital to recognize this process so you can focus on
growing forwards into motherhood. We are often bombarded with
messages about what motherhood 'should' be like, and this constant
pressure and comparison stops us from being able to define what
we want our motherhood to be like.

Motherkind Musing
- How do I feel about my identity in motherhood?
- Do I find myself wanting to go back to the old me?
- How could I be more open and curious about my emerging
  identity?

The 'should sham'

Glennon Doyle, author of *Untamed*, told me, 'The thing that really
screws us over is the picture of how we think it should be.' So often
it's not our experiences that screw us over, but the messages we've
absorbed along the way about how it 'should' be – from our own
mothers, from that mum in the Nineties soap opera you were
obsessed with, from that well-meaning but interfering aunt, and
from how women and mothers were talked about in your home
when you were growing up. That's what screws us over – when there's
a gap between how we think it 'should' be and how it actually is for
us. And in that gap, rather than recognizing that the messages are
wrong, we assume we are wrong.

The key to unscrewing yourself is to know a little bit about how
your mind works. Throughout our lives, our subconscious mind is
continually absorbing influences and information from the world
around us. I think of the subconscious mind as a vacuum cleaner

constantly running over the carpet of our lives, sucking in everything we've experienced in our lifetimes, both stuff we remember and stuff we don't. Our subconscious mind then takes all this and creates beliefs, which influence how we behave.

A belief many of us have around motherhood is that it should be easy (thanks to the media). So, the moment we start to struggle, because of, um … reality, we don't question that belief. Instead we question ourselves, telling ourselves there must be something wrong with us because this is 'meant to be easy'. But where did we get this idea from? That's our subconscious mind at work. Studies tell us that 95 per cent of behaviour is driven by our subconscious.[8,9] We have to question these beliefs so that we see what is driving our thinking and behaviour so that we can challenge our thoughts about how we think motherhood 'should' be. Let's toss these unhelpful beliefs out and replace them with the freedom to decide how we choose our version of motherhood to be.

According to Bruce H. Lipton, PhD, stem cell biologist and author of *The Biology of Belief*, we live in a subconscious state – the theta state – up to the age of seven. During these years we download our beliefs from the people close to us and our community.[10] Our first seven years, therefore, have a significant impact on how we live the rest of our lives.

I can sense you panicking about your own children – please don't. These beliefs can also be changed and updated as our brains change – a process called neuroplasticity. However, this tells us that how we experienced motherhood in our early lives has a massive impact on how we think and feel about ourselves as mothers. And – deep breath – how our children see us experiencing motherhood matters.

So what does this mean? We have to make the invisible visible, so we stop screwing ourselves over. Motherhood expert Dr Sophie Brock says to connect with the authenticity of who we are, we first have to deconstruct who it is the world expects us to be. Without digging down into the roots of the 'should sham', we find ourselves running on autopilot, downloading files of what motherhood and mothers 'should' do without pausing to think: what do I *want* my motherhood to look like? Because unfortunately our brain downloads don't automatically go through an anti-virus scanner; we have to do that ourselves.

Here are some of the common 'shoulds' I hear from the Motherkind community:

We *should* bounce back after having a baby.

We *should* have an instant rush of love for our newborn.

We *should* hold the mental load for the whole family.

We *should* have a partner.

We *should* find motherhood easy and natural.

We *should* be selfless.

We *should* work.

We *should* stay at home.

We *should* have positive feelings about motherhood – no ambivalence, boredom, or regret.

We *should* put our wants and needs away.

We *should* be more in love with our partners than ever before.

We *should* go back to work as if nothing has happened.

We *should* find parenting instinctive.

We *should* do it all, with a smile on our face.

I could write hundreds of 'shoulds' here, but what really matters is what *your* shoulds are. And each of you will have a different list based on your unique history, culture, experiences, age, race, and sexuality. But I promise you that making these invisible shoulds visible will be one of the best things you ever do. Because when you get rid of the shoulds and replace them with your wants, you'll find self-forgiveness and self-compassion, and you'll feel more confident and less guilty. I cannot tell you the freedom you will find by unearthing and unlearning the shoulds you are putting on yourself. I found so much freedom from learning that I wasn't a bad mother, I didn't mess up, and I wasn't 'not cut out for this'. I was judging myself based on unexamined ideas of what and who a mother is, which weren't even my own. Once I was able to remove the pressure of the *shoulds* and begin to think about my wants, it was the first step to becoming my own ally rather than my worst critic – a process that we'll explore in Chapter Two.

Motherkind Toolkit: What are your 'shoulds'?

Grab a piece of paper and a pen and jot down at least ten 'shoulds' about motherhood.

Then draw a line down the centre of another piece of paper and write the shoulds that are empowering you on the left, and those that are not serving you on the right. Re-write the statements on the right so they are more empowering, e.g. 'A good mother *should* have a partner' could become 'A good mother creates a loving home, whatever that looks like'.

This is a fantastic exercise to do with your partner, if you have one – what are their beliefs about what a mother 'should' do?

If you only have five minutes today …
- 'Matrescence' describes the transition into motherhood – emotional, physical, and spiritual.
- Words matter: understanding matrescence helps us to feel less alone and normalizes our experiences.
- However long you've been a mother, matrescence can offer you validation and self-compassion. The timeline doesn't matter, but acknowledgement does.
- The pressure on mothers to bounce back is immense and totally at odds with what most mothers experience.

- We can't go back to our old selves because the experience of motherhood changes us.
- When we resist this change, it causes stress and undervalues all we have been through.
- We are constantly evolving – learning to embrace and accept change frees up energy and time.
- The 'shoulds' of motherhood screw us over. When there's a gap between how we think it 'should' be and our own experiences, we blame ourselves, not the beliefs we're measuring ourselves against.
- The 'shoulds' of motherhood are deeply ingrained in our subconscious and will continue to drive our thoughts and behaviours until we make these invisible beliefs visible.
- Western society typically doesn't value the role of motherhood, and many of us don't value ourselves or the role we play.
- Change starts with us: we have to start valuing ourselves as women and mothers in order for our children to learn about their own self-worth.

Chapter Two: How to get on your own side

'There will always be someone who doesn't see your worth – just don't let it be you.'

MEL ROBBINS, AUTHOR AND SPEAKER

I'm thirteen weeks pregnant and staring at the date on the letter. I look back at the calendar again; I've missed my twelve-week scan at the hospital. 'See,' I told my husband. 'I'm going to be an awful mother, I can't even make it to the scan on the right day.' Something about growing life inside me made me harder on myself, not softer.

The truth was that back then I had no idea how to be kind to myself. I had no idea how to have my own back, how to actually like and support myself. But I knew one thing: I didn't want to pass on this toxic trait of relentless self-criticism. So, I learned everything I could about worth, self-compassion, and how to become a friend to myself. Little did I know it would be one of the most important skills I would learn, and that it would transform not only my motherhood, but my life.

Fast forward seven years and I was watching my youngest daughter trying to do a jigsaw puzzle. She was picking up each piece of the twenty in the pile, trying to get it to fit (it was painstaking to watch). Everything in me wanted to hand her the right piece, but I sat on my hands, tried not to wander off in my mind to the mess waiting for me in the kitchen, and I just kept watching. Then she started talking to herself. 'You can do it,' she said. 'I believe in you.' She kept saying it to herself, getting a little louder with every mismatched piece. She stopped and looked up: 'Why are you crying mummy?' I wanted to say, 'I'm crying because it's taken me forty years to learn to speak to myself like that. I'm crying because I've worked so hard to change my own self-talk, in the hope that it might impact yours, and it might just be working. I'm crying because no woman in my family has ever spoken to themselves like that and here you are breaking cycles (and puzzles). I'm crying because I want to believe in myself too. I'm crying because of the enormity of this moment and the mundanity of it, and I can't quite hold both.' But I thought that might be a bit much for a three-year-old, so I looked at her and I said, 'I'm crying happy tears because I'm proud of your kind words.' As self-compassion expert Dr Kristin Neff shared on the podcast, 'The more I could accept, love, and comfort myself, the more I was able to do that for my son.'

> **Motherkind Moment**
> Developing a kinder, more supportive relationship with ourselves is a gift we can pass on to our children.

The epidemic of self-criticism

If you're finding motherhood hard, that's because it is hard, not because anything is wrong with you. When I asked Olympic gold medal winner Helen Glover MBE, 'What's harder, the Olympics or motherhood?' she didn't miss a beat when she replied, 'Motherhood.'

Yet, every mother I know is hard on herself. We're already doing one of the most undervalued yet vital roles, but we make it so much harder when we criticise ourselves. We blame ourselves for not being able to manage sleep, feeding, and discipline the way the parenting books tell us we should. We blame ourselves when we feel like we can't cope, and when we're overwhelmed and exhausted. We tell ourselves we should be better at this, we should be happier, thinner, more social, and have more friends. We feel we should be better partners, daughters, sisters, and colleagues. We tell ourselves we're not doing it right, whatever 'it' is. When someone is struggling, for whatever reason, they deserve kindness – you are that someone.

However, we're relentless in our criticism of ourselves. We focus on what we've done wrong rather than the hundreds of things we're doing right. We decide that no one really likes us at the toddler group, or the school gates. We question ourselves at every turn, thinking that everyone else has it together and it's only us who feels like we're failing. I don't think it's an exaggeration to say that mothers criticising themselves is an epidemic.

This matters because negative self-talk is the single biggest block to us being able to experience more joy in motherhood.[11]

Imagine you've taken on a new project at work in an area you're not familiar with. Your boss is hovering over you saying that you should know what you're doing, you're not going to cope, and the project is too much for you. You make a small mistake (because you're human) and your boss is on you straight away telling you you're no good, you need to do better, and try harder. It would be awful, wouldn't it? You would probably burn out, stop learning, likely become anxious, and lose all your confidence. But that is what we do to ourselves in motherhood: we are learning every single day how to parent, juggle work pressures, carry the weight of the mental load, and still care for ourselves. Yet we act like that critical, mean boss to *ourselves*.

Beating yourself up doesn't work. If it did, we'd all be thriving. Shaming yourself, criticising yourself, and kicking yourself when you're down doesn't motivate you. And it definitely doesn't make you a better mother. So let's try a new way.

Start rooting for yourself

There's not much we can control in motherhood: we can't control government childcare policy, pressures from the media, whether our baby gets colic or how quickly our toddler potty trains. But we can control having our own backs through the ups and downs. We can control not piling on self-blame and criticism. We can let hard things be hard, without deciding it's our fault they are this way. We can control how we talk to ourselves. We can control whether we hate and berate ourselves through motherhood or support ourselves. Self-compassion expert Dr Kristin Neff told me that a war veteran's level of self-compassion was more predictive of whether they developed PTSD (post-traumatic stress disorder) than how much action they saw. So, it's not what you face, but how you support yourself through it that matters. When you are your own friend, you can get through (almost) anything.

A recent survey by wellbeing brand Motherly revealed that 92 per cent of the 11,000 mothers questioned felt that society does not understand or support motherhood.[12] It is without doubt one of the most important, yet undervalued, roles there is. As parents we make decisions that change lives. We shape future generations, and at times it's literally life-and-death work. So we cannot *collude* in our undervaluing. We can't gaslight ourselves into believing motherhood isn't important, vital, and hard. We have to learn to thank and support ourselves, and each other. *We have to validate ourselves.* When it's hard, when we're exhausted, when the juggle is too much, when our partners and family aren't supporting us, when we look like a mess on the outside and the inside feels even messier, when we're trying to mother and work and work on ourselves, *we have to validate ourselves.* Because sadly the chances are, no one else is going to do it for you. And even when a kind friend says, 'But you're an incredible mother, you're smashing it,' it doesn't always stick, does it? Because we don't really believe it.

Motherkind Community: Vanessa's story

'I've taken on a new perspective of myself, in that you have to be the leader of you rather than wait for others to see or appreciate you. While that would be ideal, it's important for me to appreciate myself, take care of myself, and be proud of that.'

Motherhood is never going to be all roses and plain sailing. Nothing you can do will take your problems or challenges away, because that's life, but we can learn to *support ourselves* through the challenges. We talk a lot about support systems in motherhood, so let's include ourselves in that: be your own inner support system.

There's a reason CEOs, celebrities, and elite athletes hire coaches. It's because they know that, to perform at their best, they need someone on their side, believing in them, encouraging them, and picking them up when they make a mistake. And motherhood is just as important and hard as any of these roles, so we need to become our own inner coach for what might just be the hardest challenge we'll ever face. Motivating yourself through kindness, respect, and belief works.

No one knows what it's like to be you or what your unique experience of life and motherhood has been so far. No one knows the trauma and pain you've experienced. No one knows the prejudice you've encountered or the grief and loss you've endured. No one but you knows all you've survived to be here today reading this book. Which is why you have to get on your own side. You have to start being kinder to yourself, accepting and believing in yourself. No one ever shamed and criticised themselves into being happier, and you are no exception.

This isn't just a nicer way to do motherhood; it's backed up by research. I have studied over twenty-five research papers on self-compassion, and the evidence is compelling. Being kinder to yourself has been proven to be one of the most important things you can do to improve the quality of your life.[13] Self-compassion has been proven to be one of the most powerful sources for developing healthy coping mechanisms and resilience. People who are kind to themselves are less likely to be anxious or depressed. And developing self-compassion gives you more confidence. I have thrown myself into developing a kinder relationship with myself and have experienced all of these benefits. In fact, I don't think I'd have found the confidence to write this book if I still had that critical, harsh relationship with myself.

How to become your own inner coach

I want you to think back to yourself as a baby: how perfect you were and, hopefully, how loved you were. But you hadn't achieved anything yet. You hadn't got a grade or looked a certain way or climbed the corporate ladder. And yet you loved yourself, you cried out for your needs to be met, and you took delight in your hands and feet when you first discovered them. When you were a toddler you laughed at your own jokes, demanded that things were just the way you liked them, and kissed your own reflection. You truly loved yourself.

Mel Robbins, author of *The High 5 Habit*, told me, 'When you're born, every single human being is hardwired for self-love.' So liking yourself in adulthood isn't something you need to learn for the first time – you already know how to do it. And us mothers have a shortcut, because we get to experience this again with our own children. We see them demanding our attention to watch their jump into the pool ('Mummy, watch! Mummy, watch!'). We see them love themselves, not for what they achieve but for who they are.

Motherkind Moment

Liking yourself isn't something you need to learn for the first time, it's something you need to remember – you already know how to do it.

Beliefs, thoughts, and actions

Maybe you've never seen a mother who truly believes in herself, who is on her own side, who supports herself unconditionally. If you have no map, let me give you one. I'm going to coach you through the three steps you need to finally get on your own side: *beliefs, thoughts, and actions.*

Step one: What do you believe about yourself?

Beliefs are thoughts about ourselves that we have repeated so many times that they have become our Truth (with a capital T) because we believe them, without question. Dr Nicole LePera, clinical psychologist and author of *How to Do the Work,* says that a belief is 'a practised thought'.

The other day my youngest daughter was zooming her toy train around the track laid out on the floor, while I was lost in thought about how best to explain beliefs, then I looked up and realized that the track is like our beliefs and the train our thoughts and actions. Our beliefs determine everything. What is mind-blowing about beliefs is that they operate from a subconscious level. Put bluntly, what you believe about yourself runs your life without you even *realizing* it. Beliefs tell you what you notice, focus on, how to behave. It doesn't matter what's true; it matters what you believe.

> **Motherkind Moment**
> What I believe about myself as a mother is driving my day-to-day thinking and behaviour.

It's the start of autumn as I am writing this and everywhere I look there are sticky seed pods that fall from trees and stick to my little cockapoo on our walk – each new field we venture into, a new set becomes stuck to her black fur. This is similar to our beliefs; we walk through life, picking up beliefs about ourselves unknowingly – who we are, our worth, what we deserve, and our capabilities. We're covered in sticky pods of beliefs, which dictate almost all our behaviours. So we have to pause for a moment, take a look at what we're covered in, make the invisible visible and start to peel off what doesn't serve us and replace it with new beliefs about ourselves. As neuroscientist Dr Tara Swart told me, 'If there's something that's fully submerged in your subconscious that's driving your behaviour, and you're not aware of it, you can't do anything about it unless you raise it from non conscious to conscious.'

Below are some of the beliefs I've heard from the Motherkind community:

I believe I'm not capable.
I believe that nothing works out for me.
I believe I could never be truly happy.
I believe I don't deserve my children.
I believe I could never cope on my own.

I believe I'm stupid.
I believe I'm ugly.
I believe I could never be financially free.

I have the incredible privilege in my coaching practice of seeing beneath the masks and peeking behind the curtain we present to the world. I sometimes cannot believe I have the gift to sit with a client and dive into what holds her back from getting on her own side. Sometimes, it breaks my heart. I have sat with hundreds of clients in that space of depth and truth, and as we've dived deeper and deeper I've often found that at the bottom of that ocean sits the core belief that they don't feel good enough. If you re-read the beliefs above, you'll see at the core of all of them is the belief that 'I am not good enough.' Podcast guest Roxie Nafousi, author of *Manifest*, told me, 'I really, truly believed that I was unworthy, that I was a burden to everybody and that I didn't fit in. I wasn't wanted, I wasn't liked, I wasn't loved, I wasn't accepted. And I was not enough.'

We believe that we're:
Not good enough mothers.
Not good enough friends.
Not good enough employees.
Not good enough in how we look.
Not good enough in how we live.
Not good enough in our choices.
Not good enough financially.
Not good enough just as we are.

And it breaks my heart every single time we arrive at this point, *because it's just not true.* When we don't feel good enough, we over-give, over-plan, over-worry, and over-control. Because if deep down we feel unworthy, we overcompensate in an attempt to correct this.

If deep down you don't truly value yourself, then chances are you're going to exhaust yourself trying to prove your worth as a mother. You'll put yourself at the bottom of the pile, you'll push yourself to exhaustion, and keep giving to others because you don't feel worthy of rest, support, or advocating for your needs. You'll buy your children brand new clothes and let yourself wear old, stained T-shirts that don't fit anymore. You'll buy fresh fruit for them but save none for yourself. You'll support their passions and hobbies but have none of your own. You'll make sure they always eat lunch but forget to eat yourself. You have to start believing that you are worth caring for too, and that you matter. *That you are just as important as every other member of your family.* When you live from a place of 'not enough', nothing you ever do will be good enough, for you.

From the Motherkind community:
'I've never felt good enough. I didn't understand why anyone liked me at school. I felt like I got my job by fluke, and I was going to be found out any minute. I still feel like the only reason my partner chose me was because she was desperate, and now I'm a mother, I feel like I don't deserve my children. I feel constantly worried I'm going to mess them up, so I try to make it all perfect. The pressure I put on myself is almost unbearable. I was up until 2 a.m. the other night because I wanted to handmake my daughter's costume for her nativity, not have her in a shop-bought one. I always feel like the house isn't tidy enough, that I'm not doing enough, I feel constantly paranoid at the school gates that no one likes me. I replay conversations I've had with the other parents looking for things I might have said to offend. It's taking all the joy out of my life.'

Child and family psychotherapist Louis Weinstock told me, 'You have to keep coming back to the feeling that you are enough. Constantly, we're being told, in so many different ways, especially as parents and as children, that we're not enough. We're not doing enough. We're not thin enough. We're not clever enough. We're not working hard enough. We're not self-caring enough. We're not parenting well enough. I really think the most important and simple antidote to that is to just keep coming back to this sense. And it's even a mantra that I use for myself and with my clients. Just reminding yourself, you are enough, you are enough. It's really simple.'

Motherkind Moment
Believing you are good enough is vital in motherhood, or you might break trying to prove you are.

These core beliefs are wired in us when we're young, and some psychologists believe by the age of seven. Almost everyone leaves their childhood with beliefs about themselves that aren't supportive or true. But the good news is, because of neuroplasticity (which is the brain's ability to rewire itself), we get to update these beliefs about ourselves. Much as it frustrates me when my computer reminds me that I need to update its software, we need to update ourselves too. We need a system update now that we're mothers, and that system is our beliefs.

Many of these beliefs have been passed down the generations, like a bobbly jumper, and it's our job to hold up each jumper, take a good look at it and decide if we want a new one. It's fascinating how we update our beliefs about life, about other people and the world, but rarely about ourselves. You may no longer believe in Santa, but you might still believe, deep down, that you're not good enough.

It's important to remember that these beliefs we gather about ourselves aren't a moral issue – you're not 'bad' for having these beliefs about yourself, they're just the language you learned as a child. Think about it this way: if you grew up in a household where everyone spoke French, you would speak French too. We create these beliefs based on what we see and hear around us. But we can learn new beliefs. Just like learning a new language, changing what you believe about yourself might feel clunky at the start, but step by step you'll soon become fluent in the beliefs that support and empower you.

Why are there pregnant women everywhere?

I had never really noticed that many pregnant women before I became pregnant myself, and then I saw other pregnant women everywhere. What was going on? Because I was pregnant my brain knew that pregnancy was important to me and so I was noticing all those beautiful bellies. Of course, there were just as many pregnant women before, but my brain was filtering them out because it wasn't on my agenda. It's like when you're thinking about buying a new pink jumper and suddenly you see pink jumpers everywhere. That's because you have told your brain that pink jumpers are important to you, so it scans your environment for pink jumpers. This is controlled by a part of the brain called the reticular activating system (RAS), which essentially acts as a filter for the brain. It lets in what you tell it is important, and discards everything else. And knowing about this RAS is how you can change your beliefs about yourself.

One of the core beliefs I had about myself was that I wasn't liked. It developed early on from playground experiences in primary school and stuck with me until I worked on updating my beliefs. Because I believed I wasn't liked, my brain focused (just like the pink jumper) on any time someone rolled their eyes at me, or I didn't get a reply from a friend, or I wasn't invited to a party. My brain was like a telescope zooming in on every single moment that confirmed my belief to be true.

It's no wonder that I didn't feel liked by the other women at my antenatal group. My brain, because of my belief, was looking for evidence to validate it. I was unwittingly telling my brain that not being liked was important to me. It simply wasn't noticing all the evidence that I was liked. My brain didn't register the kind smile from the mum next to me, it focused instead on the judgemental eyes from the one opposite me. It didn't notice the supportive messages from my new mum friends, it zoomed in on the one mum who didn't reply.

Beliefs are learned, so we can unlearn them

If our beliefs about ourselves are learned, then we can unlearn the ones that are harming us. Remember that a belief is just a practised thought that we have reinforced by looking for evidence that it's true. This is how we start to change our beliefs about ourselves: we look for new evidence, write ourselves a new programme, and practise different thoughts. Stop reading for a moment and look around you. Notice everything that is blue, and only look for blue. How much blue did you see? I'm guessing quite a bit. Now what did you see that was red? I bet nothing because you weren't telling your brain to look for red. But now if you look for red, you'll see it. This is RAS in action, and this is exactly what we need to do – we need to look for new updated evidence about ourselves.

Do you believe you mess everything up (maybe you even believe you're messing your children up)? Then start looking for evidence of when you get things right. 'I get the important things right' could become your new empowering belief. Start noticing every time your child is kind, loving, or calm, and allow it to sink in that you're doing an amazing job. Notice every time you get somewhere on time, or you remember to book that doctor's appointment. Notice it and let it sink in. Neuroscientist Dr Tara Swart told me, 'We can choose a new way of being, thinking, believing, by working really hard to override that natural default with this new behaviour.'

Motherkind Toolkit: Beliefs inventory

Grab a pen and notebook and answer the following:

- What are your beliefs about yourself?
- What are your beliefs about yourself as a mother, partner, friend?
- What are your beliefs about your past, present, future?

Jot down as many beliefs as you can. Try to note at least ten and make sure that some of them are positive. It may be affronting when you first do this, especially if your answers tend to be negative. If it feels too much, take a break and come back to it at a later stage, or seek support from a therapist or coach. And remember, these are just beliefs; they don't define you and they aren't your truth.

Once you have unearthed these beliefs, you need to update them into an empowering new belief and then think about what action you could take to develop this. Below are some examples from my clients.

Old belief	Where it might have come from	How this impacts my behaviour	New belief	New action
My needs don't matter	My requests and tears were often ignored or glossed over in childhood	I don't do much for me, I often let myself become exhausted or burned out	My needs matter	I will do something small for myself every day
I don't deserve for life to be easy or fun	I grew up in poverty, where we struggled every day	I don't accept any help because I feel familiar with struggle. I worry when life feels easy or fun that something awful is about to happen	I am deserving of ease and fun	I accept more help and enjoy the moments of ease
I need to be perfect	I was praised a lot for being a 'good girl' and my parents frequently seemed stressed, so I tried to be perfect	I am really hard on myself and push myself to do everything perfectly	I am good enough	I allow myself to be imperfect

As you move through your day, pause and think to yourself, 'Am I acting from an old and unhelpful belief about myself? What would I do differently if I adopted my new, positive belief?' Every action you take will either reinforce an old belief or help you to create a new one.

When I was working on changing my belief about worthiness, I worked hard every day to act from a place of worth. I asked myself, 'If I believed I was worthy, what would I do?' I'd cook myself a healthy lunch. I'd go out for a walk. I'd ask for help. I'd reach out to someone. I'd say no to that request. I'd drink more water. Acting 'as if' is an incredibly powerful tool for when you are beginning to shift your beliefs about yourself.

How to reframe your beliefs

- 'I am not good enough' becomes 'I am good enough.'
- 'I mess everything up' becomes 'I am perfectly imperfect.'
- 'I can't cope' becomes 'I can handle anything.'
- 'I am a bad mother' becomes 'I am a good enough mother.'

Repeat these throughout the day. Remember that a belief is a practised thought, so we can practise new thoughts.

Step two: *What do you think about yourself?*

Happiness expert and author of *That Little Voice in Your Head* Mo Gawdat told me, 'Thoughts and only thoughts have the single biggest impact on the state of our happiness.' The problem was that for most of my life I've lived with a critical bully in my head, and it was never louder than in motherhood. 'You're a bad mother,' I would hear. 'You shouldn't feel happy to have an afternoon without your daughter.' 'You look awful.' 'You're doing it wrong. Look at how much better that other mum is doing it.'

Motherhood turned the volume dial up on my self-critic to a hundred. Our critical inner voice becomes stronger when we do something new and when we care deeply about something. So of course in motherhood, where every day is new and our hearts have never felt so vulnerable, the inner critic is loud. And most of the time we don't even realize it's happening. It takes so much courage to show up day after day when we live with a critical voice in our heads, and I want to honour that and your ability to keep going. As Tamu Thomas, author of *Women Who Work Too Much*, told me, 'If I heard someone in the streets speaking to another the way my internal dialogue was, I would intervene.' You deserve to mother with an inner coach sitting beside you, not a voice intent on tearing you down.

Neuroscience tells us that the only way to change how we feel is by becoming aware of our inner experience and learning to befriend what is going on inside ourselves. A simple truth is that you can't change what you're not aware of, so noticing your critical thoughts is the first step to creating distance from them. According to the National Science Foundation, the average person has around 12,000 to 60,000 thoughts per day. Of those, 80 per cent are negative and 95 per cent are repetitive.[14] I find this strangely comforting, because it means we can quickly identify our repetitive negative thought patterns. Mo Gawdat, author of *Solve for Happy*, calls this repetition of negative thoughts the 'Netflix of unhappiness' – we replay scenarios as if we're bingeing on a new TV series.

Motherkind Moment
You deserve to mother with an inner coach sitting beside you, not a voice intent on tearing you down.

Motherkind Moment
We tend to repeat the same negative thoughts about ourselves – the first step to changing this pattern is to become aware of it.

Criticism is generational. Most people who are highly critical of themselves are also highly critical of others. So, if you had a critical parent who always focused on what you were doing wrong, or mocked you or was always digging at you, then chances are they were also doing that to themselves. Learning this was all the fuel I needed to want to change my inner critic for good as I really didn't want my criticism of myself to spill out into criticism of my girls. I learned from clinical psychologist Dr Nicole LePera that how we speak to our children becomes their inner voice: 'It's less the inner critic, more the inherited critic,' she told me. Psychotherapist Philippa Perry agreed when she told me, 'If we are horrible to ourselves, our kids somehow pick it up by osmosis that it's okay to be horrible to yourself.'

I want my children to have a supportive, kind inner voice, and it dawned on me that the best way I could help them develop this was to develop it in myself first. As clinical psychologist Michaela Thomas told me, 'The language you have about yourself matters because the next generation is watching you.'

Many of my clients have told me that the critical voice they hear is someone else's. They might hear their mother say, 'Who do you think you are?' or 'You can't do that.' Or their father say, 'Ha, you're working on your inner critic, what a load of mumbo jumbo.' This isn't about blaming our parents or caregivers, who were probably just passing down what had been passed to them. It's about bringing awareness to your inner thoughts, so you can begin to change them. Mel Robbins, author of *The High 5 Habit*, told me, 'When you get really in touch with the type of criticism that you're delivering to yourself, you'll realize, oh, this sounds a lot like how my dad talked to my mum, or my mum talked to herself, or my grandmother talks to my mother. And so, it's not even your voice – your brain learns patterns, and you've adopted someone else's pattern. This isn't about blame but about bringing awareness to our thoughts.'

Motherkind Community: Rachael's story

My client, Rachael, had always known she had a loud inner critic, but it wasn't until she began to write her thoughts down that she realized just how constant and ever-present her inner critic was. She wasn't sure when it first started but remembered being a worrier and feeling inadequate from a young age. Rachael recalls that after trying to become more aware of her inner critic, she noticed how all-pervasive it was – even telling her that she couldn't talk to another mum in the park because her hair wasn't as glossy as the other mum's.

> 'My mind had quickly gone to the fact that she couldn't possibly be that glamorous without plenty of wealth, a big house, and a big job, and therefore she wouldn't possibly want to talk to me. I let her child share the toys we'd brought for the sandpit, we chatted happily, and she was grateful for the toys and hoped we see each other again. Once I had the awareness, I started to see patterns in my limiting beliefs.'

Another area where Rachael lacked confidence was her career. She constantly thought that she wasn't good enough for her job. But by writing down all the evidence to the contrary, Rachael managed to reframe those beliefs. Soon it became clear that her heart was telling her that she was good enough for her job, but the real problem was that she didn't like her work. Rachael had been brought up to believe that everyone worked hard to provide for their family, so this was the route she had followed. But she now had the confidence to choose a different way to live and trust her values to guide her with the decisions she faced.

'Another breakthrough was reframing this belief to "I can provide for my family and like what I do." Previously I didn't have the belief that I was capable of anything else. In reframing what was holding me back, I became flooded with a wave of excitement for the possibilities of how I could choose to live my life.'

Motherkind Toolkit: Get to know your inner critic
To bring awareness to your inner critic, take a few moments to consider:
- Whose voice is it?
- What is the tone?
- Does it sound like your voice or someone else's?
- What does it focus on?

A thought is just a thought

How I have changed my relationship with myself, and these negative thoughts, is very simple – but it's still not easy. Put simply, I have created distance from my inner critic. Today I can hear a negative thought: 'Who are you to be writing a book?' which I hear often as I tap away. But I don't believe it to the extent that it would make me shut down my laptop and give up. I can let a thought be a thought. I can ask myself: 'Is this true? Does it serve me? Or is it just one of the random 60,000 negative thoughts I'll have today?'

Motherkind Moment

A thought only has as much power as you give it.

I don't fight with my inner critic; I don't shout back at it (there's enough sibling squabbling in my house without adding in an internal squabble between thoughts). As psychologist Dr Rick Hanson told me, 'Fighting with the inner critic is a long struggle since it wants you to start arguing with it, because then it's caught your attention. It's much better to say, "I got it, inner critic, thank you for sharing. I appreciate your efforts. I understood you a long time ago, you're not saying anything new. Thank you for sharing" and then focus on building up your inner nurturer.' One of the most powerful ways to create distance from your critic is to externalise it, to give it a voice and a name – ideally a silly one, like Mr Grinch. Then the next time you hear some version of 'you're not good enough', you can step back from that voice, and label it as coming from the inner critic, and think to yourself: 'Ah, Mr Grinch, there you go again!'

First thought, second thought, first action

An incredible tool I learned during my coaching training is called 'first thought, second thought, first action'. The theory is that our first thought can rarely change, and is likely to be critical, negative, and based on the programming we received as a child. But we can learn to change our second thought to a kinder, more supportive one and take a positive first action. That kinder voice might feel awkward and forced to begin with, and that's okay; it's a sign of how comfortable you have become with self-criticism.

Motherkind Toolkit: Reframe the critic

The next time you hear a harsh, critical thought, ask yourself:
- Is this really true?
- Does this thought support me or make things more difficult for me?
- What might a more supportive next thought be?

By doing this we can ensure our second thoughts are positive and kind.

First thought	Second thought
Why do I mess everything up?	There's also a lot I get right
She looked at me in a funny way	It's probably nothing to do with me
I upset that mum	If I did, I trust she'll discuss it with me
I can't cope	I am coping
I should know better than this	I'm doing the best I can right now
I'm a mess	Feelings are supposed to be messy
Everyone else can handle this	I have no idea how others really feel
I'm a terrible mum for shouting	I don't have to be perfect, I can repair

The most powerful words in the world are the words you say to yourself.

Trigger warning

The following text deals with intrusive thoughts. If you'd prefer not to read about this right now, turn to page 58 to skip this section.

A note on intrusive thoughts

'What would happen if I dropped her right now?' This thought was running through my head as I walked down the stairs with my newborn daughter in my arms. I still experience intrusive thoughts today and my girls are now aged seven and three. I actually 'hear' crying when I'm in the shower. I turn the water off and there's nothing but silence. Dr Caroline Boyd, author of *Mindful New Mum* and a specialist in intrusive thoughts in motherhood, told me on the podcast that these thoughts are almost 'universal' with 91 per cent of mothers experiencing them at some point.[15] 'They're part of the deal of early motherhood,' she said. 'It's part of adjusting to motherhood and the huge responsibility.'

I first had an intrusive thought when my eldest daughter was a few weeks old, and I was petrified. I thought I was losing my mind. I was sleep-deprived and had brain fog, bleeding nipples, and now intrusive thoughts. It all felt like too much and I was genuinely worried about myself. Luckily, I had learned long before motherhood to share my most feared thoughts (as fear breeds in silence), so I told a therapist friend who instantly normalized them. She was so nonchalant: 'Oh, almost every mother gets them,' she told me. I can't tell you the relief I felt, and I want to offer you that same relief now (because sadly we don't all have friends who are therapists, although: recommend). These thoughts usually fit into two categories: accidental harm or intentional harm. It can feel incredibly scary to experience intrusive thoughts, especially if they are graphic or violent.

Dr Caroline Boyd explained that 'Avoidance empowers intrusive thoughts.' The key is knowing that these thoughts are a normal part of early motherhood and not to give them too much power, as the more power we give them, the more they persist. One mum told me on the podcast that she bum-shuffled down the stairs with her baby for the first six months, because of her intrusive thoughts about dropping her. It's a counterintuitive solution: to give the thoughts less power by letting them float by in your mind and keep going with your day. Everything in me wanted to analyse and worry about the thoughts, but I now know that it's important to create distance from them.

If you are worried about intrusive thoughts, seek advice from a medical professional.

Step three: Action

Dr Kristin Neff, leading expert on self-compassion and author of *Self-Compassion: The Proven Power of Being Kind to Yourself*, told me this incredible story about how self-kindness in action helps not only us, but our children too. 'I was on a plane, and something triggered my son, and he went into a full-on screaming, flailing tantrum. I had the brilliant idea of going to the toilet, but of course it was occupied so I had nothing to fall back on except my self-compassion practice. I put all my energy onto myself. I told myself, "This is so hard, I feel so helpless," being kind to myself with my self-soothing, supportive words and holding my own hand, telling myself, "I'm here for you." I spoke to myself literally as if I were speaking to a really good friend. And when I did that, he calmed down. So, when I was agitated and overwhelmed, he would get more agitated, because he's picking up on my mind state. When I could calm and soothe myself and fill myself with a sense of kindness and care, he would calm down.'

Dr Neff defines self-compassion as 'treating yourself with the same kindness, care, understanding, when you're struggling, that you would show to a good friend. Self-compassion is one of the most powerful resources for coping and resilience we have available to us.' Learning how to be a friend to myself has transformed my mother-hood, and I have no doubt that it's also transformed my children's relationship with themselves. Watching me be a friend to myself has meant that both my girls have positive, loving relationships with themselves. And personally, I don't think there's anything more I can wish for than that. Emmy Brunner, coach and entrepreneur, told me, 'The gift of seeing your own mother nurture and love herself is an amazing thing. And so that was my pledge to myself, for me to demonstrate to my own daughters what it is to love and nurture yourself and to take care of yourself. And I feel like it is the biggest gift that I can give them.'

> **Motherkind Moment**
> Self-compassion is treating ourselves the same way we would treat a good friend.

What would you say to a good friend?

It's a truism that we are kinder to others than we are to ourselves. We find it easy to grab kind words and compassionate eyes when friends are struggling, but much harder to turn that understanding back onto ourselves. When I was coaching groups of mothers, I saw this in action almost every session. One woman was so hard on herself: 'I just can't seem to connect with my son. I'm just not cut out for this. I feel like such a failure,' she bravely shared with us. Then moments later she said these words when another mother shared a similar sentiment: 'I bet you're far more connected than you think you are. I've heard the way you talk about your daughter and there is so much love there. Perhaps you need to soften a little and let the love flow, instead of judging yourself the whole time.' I suggested that perhaps these were the words she needed to hear too, so I asked her to speak those same kind words to herself. It was a breakthrough moment for her, and as the tears flowed I could see her heart opening in front of my eyes.

Recently, I was rushing around my house mentally beating myself up. 'This house is a mess,' I said to myself. 'You're so disorganized. There's nothing for dinner. You still haven't got the laundry out of the machine; you'll need to wash it again now. And you still haven't got round to sending that birthday card. Why can't you just be ... better?' I paused, recognized this was my inner critic, took a deep breath and asked myself: 'What would I say to a friend in this situation?' The words came quickly: 'It's the summer holidays so you've got way more chores to do than normal because the girls are at home. You've got less time but you're still getting to everything that is really important. You're managing to write a book, manage your business, and still have fun with the girls. You're doing just fine, and you can all have cereal for dinner tonight.' It's such a simple tool but I love it. I am not exaggerating when I tell you I use this technique every single day. I love how we can use the innate kindness and empathy we have for others to turn even a small amount of that kindness back to ourselves.

Motherkind Community: Jennifer's story

My client Jennifer decided to get on her own side because she didn't want to pass on her inner critic to her two daughters.

'I used to be so mean to myself, in both the things I said and my actions. I spoke to myself in ways I wouldn't dream of speaking to anyone else, not even my worst enemy. I was hyper-critical of what I did. Judgemental.

Unforgiving. And it was relentless. It was like living with a bully, but one I couldn't get away from.'

Jennifer was aware that her critical inner voice had always been there and was apparent in almost every part of her life. It was especially loud around her feelings about her body and appearance. She believes this is most likely because the women around her when she was growing up were constantly berating their appearances and striving to be thinner, and she absorbed these messages as a child and teenager. The other area that Jennifer's inner critic was particularly fixated on was her performance at work. She rarely let herself have a break, even when she was exhausted.

Jennifer always thought she had to do more, do better, and prove she was good enough. She justified her approach by convincing herself that if she was better at her job, she'd be able to cope with the pressures and workload. Instead, she was exhausted, and her inner critic had eroded her confidence. But becoming a mum gave her the push to do the work needed to tame her inner critic.

'It was when I was on maternity leave with my second daughter that I knew I didn't want my girls to talk to themselves or treat themselves the way I did. I couldn't bear the thought of passing this inner critic on to my gorgeous girls. For them to feel how I did for even a single moment was unbearable. I knew I needed to learn this for myself so I could role model it for them. I'm not going to pretend it was easy to learn how to be kind and compassionate to myself after so long doing the total opposite. The easiest way I've found to access my self-compassion isn't to think of what I would say to a close friend, although I know that technique works brilliantly for many people. Instead, I like to think about what I would say to my daughters. Or what I would want them to say to themselves in a similar situation. This is how I can instantly find my most compassionate thoughts. It also makes it harder to choose the old way of thinking and doing things. Because I know that if we want something for our children, we must believe it ourselves so we can role model it.'

Now when Jennifer finds herself in a situation where her inner critic is making an appearance, she pauses and asks herself: 'What is the kindest, most compassionate choice I can make right now?'

At the beginning of this process, Jennifer thought that showing kindness to herself would make her lazy or selfish, but she has found the opposite to be true. She's now braver and bolder in going after what she wants because she knows how to support herself. She also believes the impact on her children is immeasurable.

'They [her children] have a mum who is kind to herself. A mum who can put on a swimsuit at the pool without making critical comments to the reflection in the mirror. A mum who doesn't beat herself up when she makes a mistake. They don't hear me criticise myself – so hopefully, this means they will grow up with an inner voice that is kind and supportive as well.'

Motherkind Toolkit: Hold yourself through the difficult moments

This self-compassion break is a simple thirty-second tool that I've adapted from the teachings of Dr Kristin Neff, to deal with difficult moments:

1. Awareness: Label the moment as hard: 'This is a hard moment', 'This is tough', 'Wow, this is a lot'.

2. Validation: Remind yourself there is nothing wrong with a hard moment. It's a part of life: 'Every mother has had moments like this', 'I'm not alone', 'Feeling this way is normal'.

> 3. Compassion: Show yourself the compassion you would show a close friend: 'I can handle this', 'I can get through this', 'I'm doing a good job.'

As you offer yourself compassion, you could try changing your voice to become a kind, loving parent to yourself. You could also stroke your arm or hold your own hand (this activates a calm, soothing response).

Why you will find what you look for

Psychologist Dr Rick Hanson told me that 'The brain is like Velcro for negative experiences and Teflon for positive ones.' Learning about negativity bias changed my motherhood. Until I learned that my brain was wired to look for what was wrong (which is called 'negativity bias'), I thought everything *was* wrong. The house was a mess. I wasn't achieving enough at work. The podcast wasn't growing quickly enough. My relationship wasn't supportive enough. My girls were too loud and challenging. My clothes were too old and didn't fit. I was too stressed, too disorganized, and too overwhelmed. Understanding negativity bias made me realize that because our brains are wired to focus on what is wrong, I was missing everything that was going well.

I didn't see that the kitchen was usually fairly organized, the podcast was making a huge impact and a difference to those who listened, and some of my clothes looked fantastic. I missed the moments when I felt great, when I was organized and connected to the girls, and parenting brilliantly. We've developed negativity bias because our brains are wired for survival, not happiness, and the things that are going well pose no threat. The real kicker is that by gathering up all this negative evidence about ourselves and our lives, we become more anxious and irritable. It's then more difficult for us to see the good in others, including our children. It's why when we read our children's school reports or have an appraisal at work, we fixate on the few negative comments and overlook the positives.

Motherkind Moment
You are in control of where you put your focus and energy. You can choose to focus on what you haven't done, or instead on what you have.

One night after a particularly hard day at work I was feeling irritable, distracted, and overwhelmed. I ran my daughters' bath while screaming, 'Bath time, NOW.' I sat on the damp bathmat, took a deep breath, and reminded myself about negativity bias. I looked up to see my girls' faces covered in bubbles, giggling away to each other. They were pretending to be Santa, putting on low voices and saying, 'Ho ho ho, what do you want for Christmas?' It instantly pierced my negative bubble and I breathed into the feelings of joy and love bubbling up inside me. I focused on their giggles and took in the good. So much of day-to-day life as a mother is hard work, and there is so much 'wrong' to focus on. I could have focused on why it took ten minutes of me asking for them to get in the bath, or how they hadn't brushed their teeth yet, or how much work I still had to do after they were in bed. But I countered the scales of the negativity bias by *intentionally* looking for something good. This isn't about toxic positivity or brushing over difficulties. It's about taking responsibility for how we experience our days and balancing out the positives and negatives.

Motherkind Toolkit: Take in the good

Dr Hanson taught me this simple, life-changing practice of noticing what feels good, turning up the volume on that feeling, and purposefully 'locking' it to memory.

- Note down one thing you feel you haven't done today or have 'failed' at.
- Next to it, note five things you have done today.
- Focus on your list of 'have dones', visualizing them becoming part of you like water soaking into a sponge.

I've had the privilege of speaking to many grandmothers and mothers of adult children on the podcast. They all said the same thing: they wished they'd been kinder to themselves, seen what an amazing job they were doing, and got off their own backs. Now is the time to be kinder to yourself, acknowledge that motherhood is hard and you are doing brilliantly, and be on your own side.

Motherkind Moment

Developing a positive relationship with ourselves is the foundation of an empowered motherhood.

If you only have five minutes today …
- How we speak to ourselves can make or break us.
- There is enough judgement, criticism, and lack of validation out there – we have to learn not to do this to ourselves.
- Self-criticism and blame hold us back and disempower us.
- Speaking more kindly to ourselves improves confidence, resilience, and coping skills.
- It's vital to learn how to move from inner critic to inner coach.
- We are in control of how we support ourselves through motherhood.
- Speaking harshly to ourselves is learned behaviour, and we can unlearn it.
- We are wired to like and care for ourselves, we just have to remember how to do it (see Beliefs, Thoughts, and Actions on page 41).
- Our beliefs about ourselves are formed in childhood and need to be updated in motherhood.
- The majority of our thoughts are negative and recycled.
- Learning to identify critical thoughts and create distance from them is a vital skill.
- Intrusive thoughts are common in motherhood.
- Self-compassion is the skill of being as kind to ourselves as we would be to a dear friend.
- Our brains are wired to focus on the negatives; it's our responsibility to look for the positives.
- Developing a positive relationship with ourselves is the foundation of an empowered motherhood.
- We can model to our children the skill of being on our own side.

Chapter Three: Take the pressure off

'Mothers, and parents in general, have pressures on them that are actually beyond the natural responsibility of a human being.'

DR GABOR MATÉ, INTERNATIONALLY RENOWNED SPEAKER AND AUTHOR ON TRAUMA, HEALTH AND HUMAN DEVELOPMENT

The insanity of modern motherhood is this: have a career, but don't ever miss a school play. Take care of your ageing parents, but also spend plenty of time with your children. Make sure your children do plenty of activities, but not too many. Keep on top of the life admin, but don't drop any balls. You need a village, but you must create it for yourself. And never say that motherhood is hard, because you chose this.

You know the saying 'diamonds are made under pressure'? That doesn't apply to motherhood – burnouts are made under pressure. Motherly's 2021 State of Motherhood survey found that 93 per cent of mothers reported feeling burned out.[16] And a 2023 survey by the app Peanut found that 97 per cent of mothers feel society puts pressure on women to 'do it all and be it all all'.[17] Pressure is one of the key causes of stress, so what can we do about it? Clearly a lot needs to change with how our cultural, societal, and structural systems support mothers, but you need help now. Today. And you'll find that help in this chapter. Here I'm going to focus on what psychologists call the 'locus of control', which involves working out what you can control and what you can't to help remove some of the pressure.

> **Motherkind Moment**
> If there's one thing that defines our generation of mothers, it's pressure.

Where does all the pressure come from?

There's a fascinating answer to this question, and it will change everything for you. Motherhood studies sociologist Dr Sophie Brock told me the era we are living is one of 'intensive mothering'. So, what does this mean? In her book *The Cultural Contradictions of Motherhood* Sharon Hays describes it as: '... a gendered model that advises mothers to expend a tremendous amount of time, energy, and money in raising their children'.[18] This Western ideology sprang up in the 1980s and is still going strong. Hearing this term made so much sense to me. It was a breakthrough moment for me. I hadn't previously considered the importance of understanding the water I was swimming in, the cultural soup of motherhood. I thought the pressure to be perfect, to forget myself, to give *everything* to my children, was coming just from me. But this isn't the case. Once we realize that there are immense external pressures on us as mothers, we can begin to question whether we can control these pressures, understand that we can't, and ultimately free ourselves from them. And that's what I want for you, me, and all of us: freedom from this armour of heavy pressure.

Motherkind Moment
We are living in a culture where 'intensive mothering' is seen as the parenting ideal.

Intensive mothering is the reason we put ourselves under so much pressure. It's the cultural messaging we have absorbed and internalized. It's almost as if it's in the air we breathe – and this is why we feel so guilty all the time. Our children aren't asking us to feel guilty every time we do something for ourselves, or make a mistake, or lower our standards, or have dreams, or want some space. It's the messaging we've absorbed that makes us feel guilt, and the idea that motherhood is about self-sacrifice at all costs. Dr Shefali, author of *The Conscious Parent*, told me, 'It is an inordinate amount of ridiculous, insane pressure. We are living in these nuclear families without support, raising children, trying to be professional, trying to look amazing, trying to eat healthily, trying to make money, trying to be sexy and maintain relationships. I mean, this is just insane. We are not supposed to be raising our children in these nuclear pods and overscheduling ourselves and them to insane levels.'

If we think about this pressure as the desire to meet certain societal ideals, and the 'ideal' is to be completely self-sacrificing, then of course we feel pressured. Of course we feel guilty when we look after ourselves as well as our children. Coupled with the fact that more mothers are working outside the home than ever before,[19] and it's the perfect storm. What's overlooked is that mothers today who do paid work outside of the home actually spend just as much time with their children as stay-at-home mothers did in the 1970's,[20] and that mothers typically do three times more childcare than fathers on weekdays, regardless of whether they are also working full or part time.[21] Eve Rodsky, author of *Fair Play*, told me, 'Women are still shouldering at least two-thirds of what it takes to run a home and family regardless of whether they work outside the home.'

The myth of the Supermum

It's ironic that the very idea of 'having it all' implies someone is living a full, satisfying life. But 'having it all' can mean the opposite: a pressurized, stressful life. This is known as the 'supermum myth'. Research from Bupa found that the pressure to be a 'supermum' has driven almost two-thirds of mothers to exhaustion, with one in five saying it affected their mental health. Nearly seven in ten feel guilty about taking time out for themselves, and almost half feel they don't deserve it. Where this pressure to be 'supermum' comes from is multi-layered, from our own beliefs and self-worth to the media.[22]

> **From the Motherkind community:**
> 'Society really does make a mother believe it's her fault as an individual if she's not coping and succeeding in "having it all". Finding Motherkind was my first step in realizing I wasn't alone – there were others out there finding these things tough.'

Clinical psychologist and author of *Parenting for Humans* Dr Emma Svanberg told me, 'Over the past twenty years that I've been working with parents the anxiety has risen in parents, and mothers in particular. Not only are there the day-to-day parenting challenges, but now this whole other added layer of anxiety about whether we're doing it well enough.'

It's insanity, isn't it? We're doing all this hard work of parenting and yet telling ourselves we're not good enough. It's fascinating how the increase in resources, digital courses, and social media accounts dedicated to parenting advice over the last decade hasn't reduced anxiety but increased it.

It's important to remember that we have more access to information on parenting and child development than any previous generation. New studies, online resources, and books appear almost daily telling us how vital the first five years are, how a child's brain develops, and how experiences in childhood create the blueprint for the rest of their lives. So, we have the knowledge, but we don't always have the support systems to be able to put it into practice. Which creates even more pressure. Dr Svanberg told me that this often leaves parents wanting to grab 'quick fixes, tips, and scripts', but as these one-size-fits all ideas don't always work, we risk feeling like failures.

It was never meant to be this way

For most of history we parented in small groups, with 'alloparents' (other caregivers) sharing the load. As Dr Gabor Maté, author of *The Myth of Normal*, told me, 'How we evolved was in hunter-gatherer groups. So, until a few thousand years ago, for hundreds of thousands of years of human evolution, we lived in small hunter-gatherer bands, where people lived in communities and children had multiple attachment adult figures in their lives. So, when you're living in a bungalow, or an apartment by yourself, and your spouse is off to work, and you're alone with your child and there's no one around, that's totally unnatural. Mothers, and parents in general, have pressures on them that are actually beyond the natural responsibility of a human being.'

And Lucy Jones, author of *Matrescence*, agreed when she shared her experience: 'I certainly thought that there was something wrong with me, that my particular nervous system hadn't evolved for this very intense, solo, one-on-one care without much social support. But the way we're doing it now is strange and most societies in the world do not work like this. We don't expect women to give birth, come home from the hospital – injured, probably – and then look after a baby on their own, at the most vulnerable time of their life.'

When I reflected on this it gave me so much self-compassion. It really was never meant to be this way, and we're not designed to parent and mother the way we do it in the modern world. Obviously, the reasons why we do this are largely out of our control, but seeing ourselves in this context, it's freeing. We can reframe, 'What's wrong with me? Why am I finding this so hard?' to, 'There's nothing wrong with me, and I'm finding this hard because it was never meant to be this way.'

Permission to take the pressure off

I grew up with an amazing mother, but she was also a mother who never stopped. As discussed in Chapter Two, we absorb our beliefs about how life works and our worth from the caregivers around us when we're young. Without doubt, I absorbed the message that my worth as a human is attached to how productive I am, to how much I can get done. I had been taught that the way to be happier was to do more. When I became a mother this was brought into sharp focus: as I would sit down to rest, my inner critic would say: 'There's so much to do, don't be lazy.' Almost every time I tried to take the pressure off myself, I would come up against the belief that I had to keep going no matter what. The idea that it was 'bad' to rest wasn't my own, so I knew it must be generational. And it's not just our caregivers that might have instilled this mentality in us. Amy Taylor-Kabbaz, author of *Mama Rising*, told me, 'We live in a patriarchal society that is about climbing the ladder, and achievement and focus and productivity at the expense of everything.'

> **Motherkind Moment**
> We are trained to believe that what we produce is more important than who we are. And thus, we are set up for a lifetime of pressure.

Motherkind Community: Bev's story

Bev, a Motherkind client, had always felt tremendous pressure to 'be' a certain way. Before motherhood, she would exercise most days, having convinced herself that a missed gym session would mean losing fitness. Like so many of us, Bev took impossibly high standards into motherhood. She would cook two hot meals for her son every day and take him out to activities two or even three times in-between. She was exhausted, stressed, and constantly feeling like she was failing.

A turning point for Bev was letting go of control and learning to trust herself and her capabilities. She found taking breaks throughout the day was particularly helpful in relieving the pressure (see Chapter Six for more on energy and exhaustion).

'I have always struggled to stop and take a break for fear of being lazy or not achieving. But I learned from Zoe to view a break as a "nervous system reset". My son is a very active, sensitive, and spirited boy. I realized I needed to take a break during the day to reset my system and to be calm and responsive to him. This may seem small, but it has actually been life-changing for me. It has made me better able to hold his emotions and be present for him. I have finally given myself permission to rest.'

> **Motherkind Moment**
> You are worthy, even when you're not accomplishing anything.

Learning to take the pressure off ourselves can be especially challenging when the pressurized messaging is coming at us from all angles. Taking the pressure off felt scary for me at first. Who would I be if I wasn't constantly driving myself to do more? What would happen if I dropped a few balls? Well, the world didn't end when I chose to make myself immune to the supermum pressure, and finally learned to disentangle my worth from how many things I could tick off my to-do list.

> **From the Motherkind community:**
> 'I'm so just afraid of being seen as lazy. I had a wonderful but very busy
> pressure-fuelled childhood, then a full-on pressured job – I don't think
> I know how to operate without pressure.'

Many of us live in fear that we will be seen as 'lazy'. We may have even been told we were lazy if we spent time reading, watching television, playing games, or just relaxing. This instilled the belief in us that unless we were moving, studying, or otherwise progressing towards some measurable goal, we were somehow not worthwhile. If you grew up in a household where this was the tone, you may find that your self-worth is dependent on the amount of 'work' you have completed that day. If you decide you haven't done enough, you may even lay awake at night worrying about what you didn't get done, or what you still have to do.

But here's the paradox with motherhood: so much of the work we do is invisible. There's nothing to show for it. No one sees the hour spent soothing a sad toddler, the long mornings in the park, the longer afternoons at home playing the same game over and over again. There's nothing to show for the long evenings spent researching allergies, school options, how phonics work, or how to wean. The list, and our Google histories, are endless. Not to mention the hours spent agonizing over decisions (more about that in Chapter Ten) and the 'Are they okay?' worries that swirl around our tired minds in the early hours. Our work is invisible, and there are no promotions, no salaries, and often no thanks. It's thankless yet vital, and arguably the most important work we'll ever do. As Dr Zoe Williams, general practitioner, author and television presenter, told me, 'I get far more recognition for my role as doctor than mother.'

Motherkind Moment
The invisible work of mothering is just as important as visible work.

And we have to resist the pressure because the societal messages we receive definitely don't validate our invisible, unpaid work. As founder of Pregnant Then Screwed Joeli Brearley told me, 'I would really like to see us recognize that caring for kids is work. It contributes to society. It's the most important job that anybody can do because if you really invest in your children and look after them, and nurture them and do everything that we do as mothers, you're going to create really brilliant citizens. Who are going to go on and do amazing things for the economy.'

Where do you feel the most pressure?

The first step in armouring-up against this insane pressure is to work out where *you* feel it most. Every client I've worked with has felt the pressure in different ways. Our unique histories, values, and circumstances will have a huge impact on where we feel pressure most and how equipped we are to deal with it. We all have a personal stress threshold: how much stress and pressure we can handle before we tip into overwhelm. As discussed in Chapter Two, self-awareness is always the first step towards change, because we can't change what we're not aware of. So, I'm going to help you figure out where you put yourself under too much pressure and how to change it.

When the second Covid lockdown hit I had a five-year-old and an eight-month-old. My work with Motherkind was in more demand than ever and I was deep into my matrescence. I was trying to learn how to mother two children, while also learning new ways to be with my husband, Guy, and myself. Then home schooling started. Guy had to focus on steadying his business, which was at risk of failing, so it was often just me, my business, my scared, anxious five-year-old daughter, and my beautiful new little baby. During the first lockdown my eldest wasn't yet at school, so it was easier somehow – my only task was to entertain her at home however I could. But by the second lockdown she had started primary school and the worksheets were being emailed over every day (I swear it felt like every hour).

I remember the first time I tried to home school her, the room full of optimism and coloured pens, with my younger daughter bouncing on my knee. Within five minutes both of us were crying. This is insane, I thought. She's five! What am I doing? Here we are in one of the most intense global crises we'll ever experience in our lifetime (hopefully), I'm exhausted, and yet I'm trying to teach my five-year-old to write her name. I remembered that school doesn't even start until age seven in many parts of the world. I suddenly woke up and realized that the pressure I was feeling was coming from my fear of 'What if she falls behind?'

I took a deep breath and remembered the lesson I'd learned from my podcast guests: the most important thing is how you are doing, because if you're okay, the children will be okay too. Well, I definitely wasn't okay with home schooling a five-year-old. So, during the next online lesson with our lovely teacher I explained that we wouldn't be home schooling anymore as it was just too much for me, and that I was worried the pressure might break me. Best decision I ever made. The relief was palpable. And guess what? She's now seven and can write her name just fine.

This experience gave me valuable insight that I now use in my coaching practice. Every time a client shares the pressures they are feeling, they also share their fears: 'I feel so afraid the children won't be happy, so I'm driving myself crazy trying to make everything perfect for them.' 'If we have a messy, disorganized house, what does that say about me?' 'I want to give the children more opportunities than I had, so I'm working a second job to pay for their activities.' This is the breakthrough insight we need: because once we realize that pressure is driven by fear, we can deal with the fears and give ourselves a choice. Fear is a reaction. So, once we dig a little deeper to deal with the fears, then we can give ourselves a choice to open the pressure valve.

Motherkind Moment
Pressure comes from fear. Today I will choose to trust that it will all work out.

Motherkind Toolkit: Identifying the pressure source
This is a powerful tool to help you clarify where you are putting yourself under pressure. A high score means that this is an area you often worry about, focus on, and feel pressure to get 'right'. A low score means you don't often worry or think about this. There is space at the bottom for you to add your own areas in addition to the common ones I've listed overleaf.

Give each of the following areas a rating from 1 to 10 to identify where you feel the most pressure:

1 = no pressure at all

5 = healthy pressure that feels good to you

10 = extreme pressure

Area	Score
Having a tidy, organized home	
Food and mealtimes	
Work success	
Financial security	
Education and schooling	
Health and fitness	
Self-development and cycle breaking	
Maintaining friendships	
Maintaining family relationships	
Managing the mental load	
Materialism	
Opportunities (clubs, extra-curricular activities, etc.)	
Advocating for your child's needs	
Raising happy children	
Keeping your children safe	
Other	
Other	
Other	

Focus on the areas you've given a rating of 7 or more. Ask yourself:

- Is lowering this pressure in my control?
- What is the fear driving this pressure?
- Is that fear real?

> • Is it linked to a belief (as discussed in Chapter Two)?
>
> Now ask yourself:
> • What would I do differently if I could remove the fear?
> • What is one small change I can make to take the pressure off?

What's really important to you?
From the Motherkind community:

'Somewhere along the way I had suppressed myself and my intuition and adopted the opinions of those around me.'

Freedom comes from knowing what's important to you. This knowledge is a motherhood superpower: it allows you to see what everyone else thinks is important, say to yourself, 'Good for them,' then come back to what is important to *you*. It stops you from exhausting yourself by wasting your precious time on things that really aren't that important. In ten years' time, you won't remember whether you replied to that email, if the meal was home-cooked, or that your colleague was annoyed because you left work early to go to your child's sports day. You won't remember whether your hair was washed, or if the children had matching socks, or how tidy your house was. But you will remember how you felt. This is my plea to you: stop putting yourself under pressure for things you will never remember and instead focus on what really matters to you.

However, this is easier said than done because the world invites us to do everything but focus on what matters. The moment we open our phones, or read the news, or see what everyone else is doing, we lose sight of what matters to us. It never used to be like this. We're the first generation of mothers with constant access to what celebrities feed their kids for breakfast, what activities our friend's kids are doing, and what the latest parenting fad is – all available to us with a few clicks on our phones. We have to be ruthless in our prioritization of what really matters to us. If we don't, we become vulnerable to what the world is telling us is important. Your children need this toy! You must feed your children this! Book this club! Dress your children in this! Send your children to this school! If you aren't clear what is important to you, you might find yourself feeling very, very lost.

When I feel stressed or pressured, I lose perspective. I forget what's important to me and I stress over the unimportant things. Every tiny thing starts to feel important and urgent. It's as if my mind is blind to the minutiae of life. And then my stress levels rise, my body becomes tense, and it feels like everyone is getting in the way of me having to get all these VITAL things done. The washing, replying to a message straight away, tidying the toys, knowing what we're having for dinner (at 9 a.m.), not being even five minutes late to a playdate. When I find myself stressing over little or unimportant things, it's a red flag. I know I've lost myself in the pressure of it all. If too many days in a row feel like this, life can start to feel stressful, overwhelming, and even a little pointless. So, I stop, take a deep breath, and ask myself: 'How important is it?'

Usually the answer is: 'It's not that important.' Most things in life are not emergencies. There's a big difference between the relationship you have with your kids – the love you have for them – and the job of mothering: the schedules, washing, cooking, cleaning, organizing, and planning. It's perfectly okay to love your kids but hate the job of mothering. Take the pressure off the job part and allow the love to bloom. That's the bit that actually matters. It's the love you give them that they will remember, not how tidy their room was, or whether you ironed their clothes. So in these moments I remind myself what is important to me: my connection with my girls, being kind to myself, feeling calm and content, allowing myself to feel joy, having fun, living a life in line with my values. None of those things feel urgent, but they are the most important things in my life. The moment I can helicopter above myself and regain my perspective, the stress dissolves, the panic subsides, and I feel an ease return.

Motherkind Moment

If something feels urgent, it's rarely important. If something is important, it rarely feels urgent.

Oliver Burkeman, author of *Four Thousand Weeks,* told me, 'The most freeing thing we can do with time is realize that it's finite. We can never get through all the things we want to do or that life demands of us. The way to reduce stress isn't to be more productive or efficient; it's choosing what we focus on.' Have you ever noticed how much of the content aimed at mothers out there is focused on 'helping' us do more with less? 'Helping' us be more efficient cleaners, cooks, employees? We don't need time-management tips and tricks; we need more time and less pressure. We don't need to colour code our calendars or a new way to manage the to-do list; we need fewer 'to-dos'. What if we stopped trying to do more in less time and started just doing less, or doing it less well? What if we dropped a few balls and felt okay about it? What if we could ruthlessly focus on what actually mattered to us? What if we lowered the bar? We have to say enough is enough, right now. We have to take the pressure off ourselves as if our sanity depends on it. Because it does.

Motherkind Toolkit: Take the pressure off

Ask yourself, 'What are the most important things to me right now?'
Reflect on your day-to-day pressures, to-do lists, and plans for the
next couple of weeks. Make a list of things you can:

- get rid of
- deprioritize
- ask for help with

Remind yourself:

- You can choose not to overschedule yourself. Control the things
  you can.
- You can control how much pressure you put yourself under.
- When you take the pressure off, you will feel more joy with
  your children.

An independent woman's guide to asking for help

I'm wrangling a buggy, a toddler, and a newborn, and the station
stairs looming ahead of me may as well be Mount Everest. I take
a deep breath as if to acclimatize to the altitude. 'Can I help you?'
says a kind voice behind me. 'Shall I take the buggy?' I want to say
yes. My legs and arms beg me to accept the help. What I hear myself
say is: 'I'm fine thanks.' Well, dear reader, I wasn't fine and it did feel
like Everest with no buzz at the peak, just frustration at myself.

One of my biggest areas of growth in motherhood has been
receiving support. My inner beliefs were telling me that asking for
or accepting help made me weak, and that I needed to handle it
all myself. I didn't like asking for help in case I would be perceived
as not coping or would feel indebted to other people. And I don't
need to tell you, that programme doesn't work in motherhood. Lisa
Olivera, therapist and author of *Already Enough*, told me, 'We need
to normalize that it might feel clunky and hard and uncomfortable

and awkward to receive help and care, and to even admit to ourselves that we cannot do it all.'

Tamu Thomas, author of *Women Who Work Too Much*, told me, 'I used to think: "I'm a strong Black woman, I'm an independent woman, I don't need anybody's help." But what I understand now is, I was brought up with very clear messages: that vulnerability was weakness. I used to believe that receiving was putting me in a position of vulnerability, because I conflated receiving with depending. And it's two totally different things. So that has been my biggest area of growth that has touched every area of my humanity, from friendships, romance, money, health, to acquiring knowledge. There hasn't been one area of my life that hasn't been negatively impacted by my former inability to receive. One of the greatest outcomes of this is seeing that my now-teenage daughter has the ability to state her needs and know that receiving support is normal rather than a shortcoming.'

The biggest lie we are fed as mothers is that asking for and accepting help is a weakness. In fact, it's a strength. Kate Northrup, author of *Do Less*, told me, 'Asking for help is not a sign of weakness. It's a sign of being human. And humans are herd creatures, we need each other in order to survive. And so asking for help is part of being human.' We can model to our children that asking for help is a skill and strength. Asking for help brings us closer to people, because vulnerability connects us. When I rewrote my script and realized that asking for help doesn't mean I'm not coping, but the help I receive actually enables me to cope, everything changed.

Everything is easier in my motherhood since I put down the illusionary supermum cape and started asking for help. I ask for help emotionally: 'I'm struggling, can I talk something through with you and have you just listen?' I ask practically: 'Can you do the school pick-up for me today?' And I ask informationally: 'Does your seven-year-old do this too?'

Motherkind Moment

We can unlearn that asking for help is a sign of weakness or signifies that we are not coping, and relearn that it's a strength.

Motherkind Toolkit: How to ask for help

Start small: If asking for help is new or uncomfortable, start with small requests to people you trust. Remember that any new behaviour will feel uncomfortable, and that this discomfort is a sign of growth.

Be honest: If you find asking for help difficult, say so: 'I actually find it uncomfortable to ask for help, so I'm practising asking more. Please could you help me with …'

My friend Lucy uses the phrase 'Can I make a vulnerable request?' when she is asking for help. I love this because it instantly softens the ask.

Be specific: Telling someone (or maybe shouting) 'I need more help!' isn't that helpful. The key is to be specific: state what you need help with, when, and any other details. This will also give parameters around your ask, in case the person you're asking has a tendency to over-help.

Don't overexplain: You don't need to launch into a long, rambling speech about why you need the help – this comes from a place of low confidence. Instead take a deep breath, make the request, and wait for the response.

Don't pre-empt a 'no': 'Please can you help with this, but I totally understand if it's too much or you can't, I know you're busy too.' By pre-empting a 'no' you're giving your ask less weight.

Affirmations for receiving help:
- I am worthy of accepting help.
- It is safe for me to helped.
- I open myself to the help that is available to me.

What if they say no?

One of the reasons we can resist asking for help is the fear of our request being rejected. Rejection, or hearing 'no', never feels good and if you've experienced a lot of rejection in your life, you might feel vulnerable putting yourself in that situation again. If the person you've asked for help says no, recognize your courage in asking for help in the first place. Thank yourself for your vulnerability. Then take a deep breath, especially if you feel upset or angry. It's a good idea to have a phrase ready to go, perhaps one you've practised: 'Thank you so much for being honest with me, I appreciate it. Can I ask for help again in the future?' This is a great phrase because first, you're acknowledging the honesty of the person saying no (saying no can be equally as hard as asking for help), and second, the question puts the attention back onto the other person while you gather your thoughts. The most important thing is not to take the no personally. When we say no to an ask for help it's usually because we just don't have the capacity to take the request on at that moment. The reasons are rarely to do with the person asking for help. Since I've been writing this book, I've had to say no many times when I've been asked to help, because I'm at capacity and it's my responsibility to manage my own limits (we've got a whole chapter on how to do this later, see page 217.)

Depending on what the ask is, you might want to negotiate the no. For example, if you've asked someone to help you with nursery pick-up three times a week and they say no, you could ask: 'Are you available to help at all?' They might say yes, but only once a week.

How to make things easier for yourself

Birds coast whenever they can to save precious energy, but my default position is to make things harder and more complicated for myself than I need to. The truth is, I feel more comfortable in a state of struggle and stress than I do in ease and flow. If I don't check in with myself, I tend to make too many plans, overcomplicate simple tasks, and generally make life more difficult. So now when I'm faced with a choice I'll think, 'What's the easiest option?' Sometimes even asking this question gives me enough of a pause to realize I can make it easier for myself. When my girls were younger, I used to have a 'one thing a day' rule, otherwise I'd find myself cramming in too many activities and creating unnecessary pressure. By making things easier for yourself you are taking the pressure off.

My friend never cooks dinner for her children on school days: 'They have a full, hot meal at school for lunch. They don't need a full, hot meal for dinner too. They have sandwiches. I've got an hour back every evening.' Ask yourself: What can you do to make life easier? Where can you drop the ball? Or even put the ball down? Take the pressure off.

One of my absolute favourite stories from recent years is about Marie Kondo, queen of organizing, who made a living by showing us how to live in tidy, organized spaces. She's written bestselling books, created chart-topping television shows, and has travelled the world showing us how to declutter, tidy, and 'spark joy'. She taught us how to roll our T-shirts, categorize our kitchenware, and store our Christmas decorations. Well, guess what? She had a third child and stopped tidying up. Yes, she STOPPED. 'My home is messy, but the way I am spending my time is the right way for me at this time at this stage of my life.' Here is a mother who gets it. Time is limited. Drop those balls. If Marie Kondo can give herself a break, SO CAN YOU. And maybe we could all borrow her mantra when we feel pressure: 'But does this bring me joy?' Making things easier for yourself might feel hard at first. You might even think you don't deserve it. You do.

> **Motherkind Moment**
> Ask yourself, 'How could I make this easier?'

What's your intention?

When we're learning to drive or ride a bike, we're constantly told to look in the direction we want to go, because that's where we'll end up. This also applies to setting our intentions for life. Before I pick my girls up from school, have a work meeting, meet friends for dinner, or practically anything else in my day, I ask myself: 'What is my intention?' The impact since I started doing this has been immense. Before collecting my girls I might think, 'My intention is to be present.' Before seeing friends, 'My intention is to have fun.' Before a difficult conversation, 'My intention is to be open-minded.' Before every podcast, 'My intention is to be of service, and to be vulnerable and brave.'

Motherkind client Mira was spinning out about her daughter's first birthday party. She'd had a really challenging first year of motherhood and felt this party was a chance to celebrate herself, her daughter, and how far they'd come. But she was putting way too much pressure on herself, and she was anxious about every detail. I stopped her mid-spin and asked, 'What is your intention?' 'My what?' she answered. 'How do you want to show up? How do you want it to feel?' I said. I could see her shoulders visibly dropping and her forehead softening. 'I want it to feel joyful. I want it to feel full of love and celebration. I want to be present and calm and relaxed. I want to actually enjoy the day.' Tears came as she realized that all of the stressing would probably mean that the exact opposite would happen.

Intention is incredibly powerful because it creates a shift from focusing on what you're doing to thinking about why you're doing it. And this can totally change your approach. Mira told me that as she opened her door to greet her guests, she whispered her intention to herself. 'It was as if I was a different person,' she told me. 'I was relaxed, happy, and I think it might have been one of the best days of my life.'

> **Motherkind Toolkit: Set your intention**
> Before you move on to the next task of your day, ask yourself, 'What is my intention?' Think about:
> - why you are doing this.
> - how you want to show up.
> - how you want to feel.
> - how you want others to feel around you.

Micro pressures – the little things that pile up

Micro pressures are the small things that we barely notice as we move through our day, but that build up and have an impact on us. Breaking up a sibling argument (a recent study showed that siblings argue on average every seven and a half minutes).[23] Serving breakfast in the right bowl with the right spoon. Remembering the school drop-off and pick-up times for each child. An ambiguous message from your boss. A curt message from your sister. The rejection of the meal you spent ages preparing.

We are always 'on'. Even when I'm not with my girls, I'm thinking about them. I'm ready for a call from the school or nursery. When they're sleeping, one cry and I'm bolt upright. We have to recognize the impact these micro pressures have: they are not big enough to trigger your stress response, but they stack up throughout the days, weeks, and months. A study from New York University found that micro pressures impact our working memory, our ability to keep track of what we need to get done. It can also cause brain fog (so it's not 'baby brain' making us less able to focus, but the day-to-day pressures) and make us more emotional and reactive.[24]

So, what can we do about this? The first step is awareness. Once we're aware of these micro pressures, we can work to reduce them.

'From decades of social science research, we know that a negative interaction is up to *five times* more impactful than a positive one. That means finding ways to eliminate even just a few micro stresses in your life can make a significant difference.'

ROB CROSS AND KAREN DILLON IN *The Microstress Effect,*
HARVARD BUSINESS REVIEW PRESS, 2023

Ping ping ping

One afternoon I received a message asking me if I'd like to be included in a project. It wasn't urgent. I glanced at my phone, but as I was knee deep in pasta pesto and tense negotiations about which spoon was the 'right' one, I didn't reply straight away. Another message came through thirty minutes later: 'Hello?? Do you want to be involved or not??' it said. This is a perfect example of a micro pressure. We live in a world of instancy where the average response time to a WhatsApp message is less than one minute.[25]

In 2019 I co-commissioned a study to understand the impact of social media on motherhood. We found that on average, since becoming parents, mothers spend an *additional* three hours and twelve minutes online each day.[26] Of course we do; often this is a time without much adult interaction and so many unknowns, so we turn to Google for answers. But we need to understand the impact of this so we can make small tweaks to protect our state of mind. Sometimes I open my social media apps and I feel like I'm being screamed at by a million voices. And that's because I am. On Instagram alone, 95 million messages are posted every single day.[27] So many of us (me included) open up our phones on the loo or while the pasta is cooking, for a quick brain break. But it actually achieves the opposite. Study after study shows that social media impacts anxiety, depression, and sleep. But why? It all comes down to the feel-good chemical dopamine. Laughing at a funny meme, liking your mate's post, having them write 'so gorgeous' on the pic of your toddler in the park, all cause us to release dopamine. It feels good, right? But what goes up must come down as our brains are always trying to rebalance. So, after the dopamine hit, our levels drop, which can feel like a comedown. Have you ever been scrolling at bedtime, and you know you want to put your phone down, but you just can't seem to stop? That's the dopamine crash in action. It's become addictive.[28] The moment you're aware of this, you've taken back some of the power.

I need strict rules with my phone and social media, because without a doubt I have been addicted to it at times. It's important to remember that if you find yourself scrolling way more than you want to, it's not your fault; social media is designed to be addictive (as demonstrated by the docu-drama *The Social Dilemma*) and we aren't designed to take in the amount of information it subjects us to. We have the exact same brains as when we lived in small communities of fifty people, when the only knowledge we had was passed down to us by people we knew.

Motherkind Moment

Our phones and social media are a constant micro pressure that we need to mindfully manage.

Motherkind Toolkit: Reduce the micro pressures

As you go through your day, think about any micro pressures you could reduce. Some of mine include:

- Not arguing about coats and shoes every time we leave the house (they go in my bag for when they are inevitably requested five minutes later).
- Laying out options for cutlery at the start of a meal.
- Putting my phone in another room when I'm with my daughters, and muting all notifications.
- Laying out school uniforms and sports kits the night before.
- Not taking a call when I'm in the middle of something.

The mental load

The dishwasher needs salt.

Have I got a present for the birthday party this weekend?

When is parents evening? Have I missed the booking deadline?

Have the girls eaten enough vegetables this week?

I didn't miss my niece's birthday, did I?

We need to shop for groceries.

What are we going to eat tonight?

I need to go to the shops before picking the girls up.

I need to book that allergy test.

Have I spoken to my best friend this week?

What uniform do they need tomorrow?

Have I filled out that form?

Have I replied to that email?

That mum asked about a playdate, I still haven't replied. I bet she thinks I'm rude.

When did the girls last go to the dentist?

I need to sort through the girls' clothes.

What are we doing for Christmas?

Did I pay for the girls' swimming lessons?

My daughter asked me about dance lessons, I still haven't researched that.

Are the girls doing okay?

When was the last time I called my mum?

The toys are a mess again, why can't I keep on top of them?

The freezer needs defrosting.

I haven't vacuumed all week.

We need loo roll.

What time is pick-up today?

Do I have snacks ready to take?

Remember, they don't like those snacks.

Am I too soft with them?

Should I just take any snack and let them deal with it?

No, I'll take the snacks they like.

Where are they again?

Found them, better go.

Where are my keys?

Oh no, I'm late …

All of the above is on my mind as I get ready to pick the girls up from school. This is a snapshot, but this mental ticker tape is pretty much constant. It's called the mental load.

> **Motherkind Moment**
> The mental load is the invisible work it takes to manage a household and a family.

It's thinking of all the things. It's the planning ahead and project management of family life so it can keep going. And it's exhausting. Just as with matrescence, understanding this made me realize I wasn't failing, and I wasn't crazy: it was the mental load. I remember the relief when I first understood it wasn't just me who had the unrelenting low-level whisper of to-dos and not-dones constantly running through my mind. But it isn't just the tasks that need to be done, it's the pressure and worry that comes with them.

I remember the first time I organized a playdate. It wasn't just the time taken to plan and organize the day, it was the constant questioning of myself that I found most exhausting. Is it okay to have them over and not offer lunch? What if the little girl is scared of our dog? Will the other parent judge how messy the toys are? How long should a playdate last? The mental load isn't *just* the thinking and the doing – it's the worrying about the thinking and the doing as well. It's the mental load, squared.

The hardest thing about the mental load is that it never ends. You will never get to the end of the to-do list and there is no break from it (even a blissful childfree afternoon is often spent catching up on the family to-do list). It's constant. In the UK women do about 60 per cent more unpaid work than men, according to the Office for National Statistics.[29] The world of work is unrecognizable for women compared to a hundred years ago, but have things really changed that much within the home? As psychologist Dr Rick Hanson told me, 'We have mothers who are taking advantage of long-overdue opportunities in the workplace, but without any real reduction in their load at home, so that has not changed very much, probably since my own parents time.' Joeli Brearley, founder of Pregnant Then Screwed, told me, 'We do have shared parental leave. It's a system that makes no sense whatsoever. It's really complex, and most people don't understand it. Only a small percentage of families are even eligible for shared parental leave because of the way it's set up; the most recent data shows that only about 2 per cent of families even use it. So, it tends to be the mothers that take the time off.'

It's often during maternity leave that this inequality in heterosexual relationships is set up. Before we had children both my husband and I worked full-time, and things at home were equal. We both planned and cooked meals, we both did laundry, and planned weekends away and nights out. He managed his family commitments, and I managed mine. It was when I took a break from paid work after our first child was born that it all changed, because I was 'at home'. I naturally started picking up all the home-related tasks and before I knew it, I was doing the majority of the meal planning, cooking, washing, organizing family visits, booking medical appointments, and everything else that goes into running a home. When it was time for me to go back to work, I took the lead on arranging childcare. I researched options, interviewed childminders and nannies, and visited nurseries. And just like that the household responsibilities started to become uneven. Luckily, there's an incredible system to redress the balance, if you need to.

Fair Play

Eve Rodsky, author of *Fair Play*, told me that she asked herself: 'How did I become the default for literally every single childcare and household task for my family?' This question drove Eve's passion for making things more equitable within the home. Eve realized she had become the 'she-fault' parent and worked for seven years to devise a system to make things fairer. Her Fair Play system comprises a hundred cards, each representing a different area of family responsibility. How you divide up the tasks will, of course, be completely different for every family, and Eve says it's 'rarely 50:50', but the most important thing is that when you own a task, you own it completely – conception, planning, and execution.

For example, knowing that your daughter's best friend is dairy intolerant (conception) so you'll need dairy-free milk for the playdate (planning) and then going out to the shops to buy it (execution). Eve told me that often women do the conception and planning, and then ask for support with the execution, but 'If I have to ask you, it's not helpful to me.' It's the mental space (the executive functioning, as it's known) that we need to reduce. Real freedom comes from not having to think about it at all.

The first time I experienced this was when Guy took full ownership of our daughter's sports activities: he chose the class, booked and paid for the sessions, took her to training, bought the kit, made sure the kit was washed and ready each week, remembered to pack a snack and water bottle, emailed when she couldn't make it, and handled it with her when she wanted to stop going. Eve told me that partners (usually men) say they feel happier once the tasks are divided up because there are fewer resentments, fewer arguments, and studies show even more sex.

How to redress the balance

Make the invisible visible

The first step is to make the mental load visible. You can use Eve's Fair Play cards or make your own list of everything you do to run your home and family. If you have a partner or co-parent, you can then start the conversations about how you'd like to share the load more equally. If you're a single parent, you can discuss this with your support network or other people in your life who might be able to share the load with you. You may never have experienced inequality with the mental load or you might be happy with your current set-up – I still invite you to make the invisible visible by capturing all you do, as it will give you a new perspective on how much you're holding.

Start the conversation

Eve explained that most women are already communicating about the mental load with their partners, through eye-rolling, resentments, snapping, shouting, or distancing, so it's 'not a conversation start, it's a conversation shift'. It's not an easy conversation to have, so it's important to choose a time that is going to work for you both and agree this beforehand; this isn't the kind of conversation you want to have on the spur of the moment or mid-argument. You need to be feeling calm and grounded. Think about what you want to get out of the conversation and how you're going to communicate this. It could be that you use the Fair Play card deck or suggest working together on a spreadsheet where all the tasks are listed and shared (this is what we did).

When training to be a coach I learned the skill of the 'open question', where instead of saying, 'We need to do this,' you ask: 'How can we work together to achieve this?' It sounds obvious but it makes a big difference because it implies respect and an open mind to work together. There is no hierarchy – you're not the expert with all the answers, and you aren't dictating. You're a team. If we feel accused of something we can quickly become defensive and focus on putting our point across, rather than hearing the other person or solving the problem.

A huge shift in communication with my husband came when I realized that it wasn't me versus him, it was us versus the problem of the mental load. It kept us on the same side, as a team, rather than adversaries. There are sadly many relationships that don't work as a team, or worse still, your partner might not care about you holding all the load. I would recommend reading Eve's *Fair Play* book, which covers these challenges and more.

Motherkind Toolkit: How to have the mental load conversation with your partner
- Avoid accusations, anger, or confrontation – the other person will likely have a stress response, and this probably won't lead to a constructive conversation.
- Use 'I' rather than 'you' statements, e.g. 'I feel really overwhelmed with having to manage everything,' rather than 'You don't do enough.'

- Make observations rather than accusations, e.g. 'I notice that I do all the school admin; have you noticed that too?'
- Say how you feel, rather than how the other person makes you feel.
- State what you want to happen, e.g. 'I'd like us to find a different way of dividing up the tasks of running our family. Are you open to that?'
- Lead with curiosity over criticism, e.g. 'I wonder how we could work together to figure this out?'

If you only have five minutes today ...
- If there is one thing that defines our generation of mothers, it's pressure.
- In one survey, 94 per cent of mothers said they feel burned out and 97 per cent feel the pressure to 'do it all and be it all'.[30]
- We are living in an era known as 'intensive mothering' where the cultural ideal is mothers who give 'everything' to their children.
- Understanding cultural and societal pressures is vital and empowers us to change how we respond to these pressures.
- This external pressure, coupled with more mothers working than ever before, creates a perfect storm of pressure.
- Anxiety felt by mothers is at an all-time high.
- We are not programmed to parent in isolation; we are designed to raise children in small groups with many other involved caregivers (alloparents).
- We need to learn to resist this perfect storm, by taking the pressure off ourselves.
- Your worth is not based on how much you're able to do or achieve.
- Much of the work of mothering is invisible, so we can put ourselves under pressure to achieve 'visible' successes.

- The key to reducing the pressure on yourself is to work out where you feel it.
- We all have a different capacity for how much pressure we can handle.
- Pressure is driven by fear, so once we understand what fear is underlying the pressure, we can work to ease the pressure.
- Working out what is really important to you is a superpower, because it enables you to stop worrying about things that don't really matter to you.
- Asking yourself 'How important is it?' is a brilliant perspective-changer if you find yourself getting lost in the little stresses of the day.
- If something feels urgent it's rarely important; if it feels important, it's rarely urgent.
- Asking for help is a skill we have to develop and it's a strength, not a weakness.
- We have the power to make things easier, not harder for ourselves.
- Focusing on our intention is a simple way to take the pressure off and focus on what is important.
- Micro pressures are the little day-to-day stresses that build up to have a big impact.
- Our phones are one of the biggest micro pressures, and we need to learn how to manage them, rather than having the phone manage us.
- The mental load is the invisible work it takes to run a family and household.
- The 'Fair Play' system can be used to discuss and implement more equality in domestic and care tasks.

Chapter Four: Perfect doesn't exist

'I can be an imperfect human and my children will still thrive.'
DR JULIE SMITH, CLINICAL PSYCHOLOGIST AND AUTHOR OF
Why Has Nobody Told Me This Before?

I hate perfectionism in motherhood. I hate how it makes us feel like we're not good enough. I hate how it makes us wear a mask to give the illusion that we're fine, even when we're on our knees. I hate how it stops us asking for help. I want to be the perfect parent, because I want my girls to be okay. It comes from such a loving place; the destination is right, but it's the wrong route. Trying to be perfect isn't going to help our children – it's going to give them a mother who is stressed out, exhausted, self-critical, and probably not okay.

It was breastfeeding that nearly broke me. I dreamt of long days with my heavenly-smelling newborn nuzzling at my breast. The reality couldn't have been more different. The latch wasn't right and I would cry when my baby girl woke up because I knew I'd have to try and feed her. I got mastitis and I bled, but I wouldn't give up. 'I will not fail at this,' I thought to myself. I was not about to let something as ridiculous as the reality of the situation get in the way of my vision of perfect breastfeeding. When she latched on, it felt like shards of glass cutting through my nipple as her little mouth started to suck. Such was my focus on successful breastfeeding that I would pump after every feed so she could have breastmilk even when we were giving her a bottle. As I result, I was always either feeding, pumping, or cleaning the pump and bottles. I couldn't see that perfectionism was driving me into the ground.

By the time my second daughter was born my perfectionism was firmly in check and we combined breastfeeding with formula from day one, and then she was formula fed from six weeks. I can't tell you the difference it made to my mental health. This story isn't about breast versus bottle (could I have chosen a more contentious topic?); it's about perfectionism, and how in motherhood it can break us. Feeding my daughters wasn't something I could get an 'A' grade in. Working hard wasn't going to get me through, and it wasn't something I could control. The experience taught me that perfectionism and control (two of my most loved coping behaviours) weren't going to work, and I had to find a new way.

Motherkind Moment
Perfectionism makes the already hard job of mothering almost impossible.

If I had a magic wand, there are many wishes I would make for you, and one of them would be to take perfectionism away in motherhood. Perfectionism will screw you over because motherhood is so inherently imperfect. Our children are so unpredictable, so messy, and there is so much for us to hold, to do, to be, that it's impossible to do it any other way than imperfectly. We have to learn to take our days as they come and let go of any expectations and illusion that we can control every detail of our lives. Michaela Thomas, clinical psychologist, told me, 'When the pressure to perform comes from both our internal mindset and external pressure, to be the "perfect" mother, then those two pressures combined create the perfect storm for burnout.'

Perfectionism is misunderstood

'There's no way I could be a perfectionist,' a client told me. 'I'm far too imperfect.' Perfectionism is misunderstood. Many of my clients have rejected the idea that they are perfectionists: 'I don't achieve enough,' they tell me. You can be a perfectionist and have a messy house. You can be a perfectionist and never arrive anywhere on time. You can be a perfectionist and regularly drop balls. Perfectionism isn't about being perfect, it's about *trying* to be perfect.

Perfectionism is when we struggle to accept ourselves as we are. It's a way of thinking that makes us strive for impossibly high standards and never be satisfied with what we've achieved. Perfectionism is like a mirage as it keeps us striving towards some perfect end point that doesn't exist. Even if we arrive, sweaty and tired, at something close to perfect, we still don't think it's good enough. So the end point disappears, and we keep running on to the next thing. It's like a cruel hamster wheel – it just keeps on going and there is no end in sight. Michaela Thomas continued, 'Perfectionism is a constant pursuit, a constant striving for high standards that are impossible to meet but yet we keep trying. So it's not the destination, it's the pursuit that is the problem – that is the thing that robs you of both your energy and your joy.'

> **Motherkind Moment**
> Perfectionism is a way of thinking. It makes us strive for impossibly high standards while never feeling satisfied with what we've achieved.

Where does perfectionism come from?

We aren't born perfectionists. Our babies don't obsess over the perfect way to form their first smile or take their first steps, they just do it. Our toddlers don't worry about the perfect way to jump in the puddle, they just go for it. Our pre-schoolers don't decide their day is ruined when they drop their lunch on the floor, they just get on with it (and maybe just make the floor their plate). Perfectionism is a learned response to the environment around us; it's what psychologists call 'adaptive'. We have adapted to the environment around us and developed a set of behaviours to help us feel accepted.

Clients in my coaching practice who struggle with perfectionism often had critical parents or caregivers, or have been in environments with unrealistic standards or too much focus on results and success. We are wired for connection and attention, so if as children we felt more connected or were given more attention for being 'good' or 'successful', then this behaviour will have become part of our belief system.[31] As children we don't question the environment; instead, we question ourselves. It's like being the tiny doll in the middle of a set of Russian dolls: layer after layer of behaviours and ways of being in the world are added to protect us in the middle.

Motherkind Musing
Which of the following common traits of perfectionism in motherhood do you relate to?

- Holding yourself to unrealistic expectations: you set extremely high and unattainable standards for yourself as a parent.

- Fear of getting it 'wrong': you might have a deep fear of making mistakes or falling short of your own expectations.

- Constant need for external validation: perfectionism means you rarely feel good about yourself, so you will seek validation from others.

- Finding it hard to ask for help: that perfectionist voice tells you that you should be able to handle it all alone and that others wouldn't do it right anyway.

- Too hard on yourself: perfectionism comes hand in hand with self-criticism and guilt.

- High levels of stress and anxiety: because the pressure to meet unrelenting standards is overwhelming.

- Low self-esteem: you struggle to value yourself and feel enough, because there is always something else you should be doing.

- Never celebrate yourself: you put so much pressure on yourself to be perfect that you can't enjoy any of your achievements.

- Finding it hard to make decisions: you believe there is a 'right' way to do things so you often procrastinate and leave the decision making to the last minute, then change your mind.

- Don't trust yourself: often asking others about your decisions and choices.

- Holding other people to too high standards: and/or are overly critical of others.

- Ensuring that things look good on the outside: wearing a mask, rarely being vulnerable or allowing others to see the messy side of your life.

- All-or-nothing thinking: you have a tendency to see a situation as either black or white, or right or wrong.

When we don't feel good enough

'When perfectionism is driving, shame is always riding shotgun. And shame, at its core, is not feeling good enough.'

BRENÉ BROWN IN
The Gifts of Imperfection

When we dig down to its roots, we realize that perfectionism is a fear of disapproval and of not being good enough. In Chapter Two we discussed how our beliefs drive our behaviour. Well, I have never felt good enough. I didn't feel good enough to be in the 'cool' gang at school. I didn't feel good enough to have the wonderful friends that loved me at university. I didn't feel good enough to have landed a good graduate job. And I didn't feel good enough for my children. Nothing I did was ever good enough for me. So I over-compensated, worked harder, gave more, and pushed through.

> **Motherkind Moment**
> Perfectionism is a fear of disapproval and of not being good enough.

For a long time, I believed my inner voice when it told me: 'You can't get anything right.' I believed it when it told me I was a 'bad' mother for not being able to breastfeed, that I was going to 'mess up' my girls when I struggled to be present with them. Mel Robbins, author of *The High 5 Habit*, agreed when she told me, 'I looked in the mirror every morning, and I saw a woman who had not done enough. So many of us are struggling with perfectionism because we don't believe that we are worthy as we are. Women, in particular, equate our self-worth, and whether we're deserving of love, with being perfect. Having the perfect hair, the best make-up, the best birthday party, the best-looking marriage on social media … we believe that it's not until we achieve that thing that we are worthy of being loved or celebrated.'

Messages of perfectionism are tricks because we can never achieve their goals. We cannot feel good about ourselves or what we have done while these messages are driving us. We will never be good enough until we change the messages and tell ourselves we are good enough NOW, then we can start approving of and accepting ourselves. We are allowed to be good-enough mothers.

A note on comparison

Social media is an incredible place to hang out as a mother; you can find connection, expertise, ideas, support, friendship, and validation. It's also a terrible place to hang out as a mother, as we can receive judgement, comparison, envy, confusion, and information overload. I couldn't write about perfectionism in motherhood without talking about social media. In many ways I love social media – it has enabled me to reach millions of mothers with my message and connect with the most incredible community. Perhaps you're even reading this book because of social media.

But there is no doubt that it also increases feelings of 'not enoughness' and comparison. In 2019 I co-commissioned a study about perfectionism in motherhood. We spoke to 1,000 UK-based mothers of all demographics and a very clear picture emerged that social media makes mothers feel pressure to be 'perfect'.[32]

Motherkind Moment
We are the first generation of mothers raising our children with social media.

None of us knows what we're doing with social media. New studies on the impact of social media emerge almost as quickly as new apps appear, and we're really all just learning as we go. It seems crazy that we can open an app on our phone seeking connection, and the first thing we might see is a beautiful mum taking her equally perfect daughter out for an expensive day trip, when at the same time we're cooking the kids pasta pesto (again) with messy hair, messy kids, and no day trips whatsoever on the horizon. It's no wonder we start to compare. Social media is comparison on steroids.

Of course, we consciously know that we're comparing our behind-the-scenes to someone else's curated reel, but our subconscious brain doesn't recognize that, and it goes straight to comparison. Our brains are simply not designed to handle that amount of information, and they aren't designed to handle Instagram. Our brains are wired to compare; in fact, our brains are scanning and comparing all the time without us even realizing it. Comparison is human nature, and it starts early on in life. But you don't need to tell us mums that – how many times has your toddler been happily playing with a toy car, then another child comes along with a bike and suddenly they want the bike? It's innate. So it's absolutely not your fault if you find yourself in a scroll hole, feeling less than and lacking, but it is our responsibility to do something about it.

I have struggled so much with social media comparison that I developed a golden rule for myself around it: if I'm feeling low or insecure I won't go on. It sounds extreme but when I tried the 'Remember: it's just a highlight reel' thought, my conscious brain wasn't processing it quickly enough, and I would still come away feeling worse about myself. I won't patronize you with obvious advice like 'curate your feed' because my feed is only full of kind, inspiring, wise people, and if I'm feeling wobbly it will still leave me feeling worse about myself. Even a picture of someone sharing how messy their morning has been can leave me feeling worse if I'm in a state of perfectionism. I've learned the hard way that it is better for me to message a friend for connection rather than open a social media app. On a good day (or hour) when my perfectionism is in check, I feel good enough, secure, and I love social media. I love sharing the Motherkind message. It's not the thing that's the problem, it's how you use the thing.

Motherkind Musing
- How does comparison feed into my perfectionism?
- Do I need to create some boundaries for myself with social media?

Good enough is just perfect

Perfectionism doesn't let you see what you *are* doing. Good enough is never good enough. You may have got your children dressed, fed, and at school on time, but your perfectionism won't let you celebrate that – it will tell you that you should have also replied to that email, unloaded the dishwasher, been more friendly to that mum at the gate, said something different to the teacher. Perfectionism erases what you have done, and only makes you see what you haven't.

Perfectionism makes us think in black and white: we're a good or bad mother. But nothing in life is binary, especially not motherhood. It's a skill to be able to mix the black and white together and live in the grey.

Motherkind Moment
I'm good enough. Sometimes I nail it, sometimes it's awful. And that's okay. That's life.

Motherkind Moment
Perfectionism is like windscreen wipers for your achievements – it instantly wipes them away and tells you to 'do more'.

As psychologist Dr Rick Hanson told me, 'A mother is like a decathlete with ten events (actually, more like a hundred). You may not be the best in the world at any single event, but you can be more than good enough at all of them together as a package. That's how to judge yourself.'

Perfectionism is a trait that becomes evident in early childhood. I remember when my eldest daughter was four, she screwed up a drawing in anger because she'd made a mistake. That was all the fuel I needed. Perfectionism is handed down from generation to generation, and I wasn't about to allow it to infect the next one without putting up a fight. So, I started making mistakes loudly. I'd tell her about the mistake I made at work that day and how I handled it. I made sure when I dropped something I didn't say, 'What's wrong with me?' Instead, I'd say, 'Oh, doesn't matter.' I was on an imperfection mission. A couple of months ago my eldest daughter, now seven, messed up her homework. 'Uh oh, doesn't matter,' she said. 'I can just try again.'

You get to decide

Releasing yourself from the shackles of perfectionism isn't about giving up: it's quite the opposite. Shaking off my perfectionism has freed up so much energy that I've achieved more in the past couple of years than during the preceding decades. Allowing myself to get it wrong, to mess up, to try and try again, has meant I've been able to imperfectly write this book, imperfectly grow the Motherkind platform, imperfectly become a more and more attuned and present mother, imperfectly change the dynamics in my marriage, imperfectly train for a marathon (which I eventually dropped out of because ... imperfect). I'm not saying any of this to show off, but to show you what is possible when we give ourselves a break, dive in, give ourselves permission to be messy. Knowing I can try something new with my girls and feel okay if it doesn't work out the way I'd planned means I'm able to do more, not less. There is such a freedom in knowing you have your own back. With this freedom, you get to decide what is good enough for you and your family. Maybe in some areas you need to lower the bar more; maybe in some areas you want to hold yourself to a higher standard. Free from that critical, perfectionist inner voice, you get to decide.

Motherkind Musing
- Where are your standards and expectations of yourself too high?
- In what situations does your critical, perfectionist inner voice become loudest?
- What would 'good enough' look like for you?

Motherkind Toolkit: Reminders for imperfection
Remind yourself:
- You are allowed to be an imperfect parent.
- Messing up is part of life.
- Aim for progress, not perfection.
- You are worthy of love.
- You can be good enough.

Focus on how things feel, not how they look

Last Christmas I decided that I would only focus on how the day *felt*, not on how it *looked*. I decided that I would take the pressure off trying to create the perfect family Christmas and take time to actually enjoy it. I let go of the timings and should-dos and had fun instead of peeling potatoes. I let the wrapping paper linger for hours on the floor while we played with new toys. We laughed and we were happy inside but messy outside. That's the right way round. What would happen if we focused more on how we feel, over how it all looks? What is the point of a motherhood that looks perfect on the outside but feels constrained, intense, and pressured on the inside?

Motherkind Toolkit: Reframe decision making

For just one day practise making decisions based on how it feels over how it looks.

Notice what different decisions you make and how you feel at the end of the day.

Allow yourself to be 'good enough'

I was recently asked by a journalist about my favourite part of hosting the *Motherkind* podcast. I think my answer surprised her. The most enriching part of speaking to world-leading experts isn't the knowledge I gain, it's the permission. Let me explain.

Dr Becky, founder of Good Inside, is one of the leading voices in parenting right now and has been called the 'millennial parenting whisperer' by *TIME* magazine. She told me, 'I get it wrong all the time. I actually have to watch my own workshops sometimes because in my parenting I'm not Dr Becky at all; I'm Becky, a struggling mum.' A permission slip to be imperfect. Dr Shefali, author of *The Conscious*

Parent and Oprah's favourite parenting expert, told me about how she messes up all the time. She actually started to focus on parenting in her psychology practice because she found it so unbelievably hard: 'I don't want people to think that I'm some Zen monk here who never loses her shit. I lose it all the time.' A permission slip to be imperfect.

Dr Gabor Maté, internationally renowned speaker and author on trauma, health, and human development, shared with me how wrong he'd got the early years of parenting. How unavailable he'd been, how imperfect. A permission slip to be imperfect. In fact, as I sit here mentally scanning the hundreds of experts I've spoken to, almost all of them have told me how they mess it up and get it wrong. So we can give ourselves permission to mess up too.

The 'good enough' parenting concept was developed by Dr Donald Winnicott in the 1950s. Winnicott found that meeting a child's needs just 30 per cent of the time is sufficient to create happy, well-attached children. And that doing so boosts their resilience.[33] That's right – three out of ten is really ten out of ten.

Psychologist Dr Maryhan Baker told me how we do our children a disservice by trying to be perfect and get it right all the time, because that's not how resilience is developed. What if it's good when we make mistakes, because by doing so we give our children permission to make their own? When we model repair, we show our children how they, too, can repair. When we forgive ourselves for being imperfect, we show our children that they, too, can be imperfect. And isn't this really what we want for our children, to allow them to be fully themselves? Imagine if we could (imperfectly) model that. Wouldn't the world be a different place?

Motherkind Moment

When we model imperfection to our children, we allow them to also show up as their own imperfect, authentic little selves.

Celebrate the small things

I have a wonderful friend who always asks me, 'And how are you going to celebrate that?' When I got my first million downloads on the podcast, I was thrilled for a moment, then my thinking quickly went back to the day-to-day tasks. It was only when my friend asked me that question that I realized this milestone represented hundreds of hours of work and countless hurdles overcome. So, I celebrated and it felt so good to take a moment to recognize the achievement.

We're so busy running from one thing to the next, but if we're not pausing to celebrate the wins, what's the point? Celebrations don't just need to be for the big things – when we celebrate the small things, we give ourselves a sense of daily accomplishment. It's likely no one else is going to notice or celebrate these small moments, but you can. You can take responsibility for noticing all the little things you do. Think about the last week alone: I bet you've had at least ten small wins. Cooked a dinner everyone ate? Set a boundary? Said no? Did something different? Remembered all the kit? Asked for help? Got to bed on time? Had a moment of joy with your children? These small wins matter – they are the threads that make up the fabric of your life. Even if you don't think you deserve it, celebrate anyway.

Motherkind Toolkit: What did you do today?

One day this week, jot down everything you do in a day, from the moment you wake up to the time you go to bed. You'll be amazed at how much you are achieving.

Mess up and repair

Dr Becky, founder of Good Inside, says that repair is 'The single most important parenting strategy we have.' Why? Because we all mess up. Of course we do, we're human. We don't need to be perfect; we need to learn the skill of repair.

Messing up is part of parenting and life in general. It's especially part of parenting if we're trying to break cycles. If we don't have a blueprint for the type of mother we want to be, then how on earth are we supposed to learn? The answer is, we learn by messing up and repairing. The challenge is that most of us didn't have this modelled to us because repairing with children just wasn't a feature of past parenting. So this is a skill we have to learn. Saying sorry to our children doesn't make us weak, it doesn't give our power away. In fact, it does the opposite; it builds love and connection. And Dr Becky believes that 'What defines us is not whether we mess up, it's what happens after.'

My eldest daughter wanted to climb a tree. 'Go for it,' I said. She got to the top, climbed halfway down, and started panicking that she was stuck. 'Mummy, help me!' she wailed. I thought she could handle it and I'm working on growing her confidence, especially physically. 'You can do it,' I said firmly. I refused to help her. After a lot of protesting she tried to get down. Well, dear reader, it did not go well. She flailed out of the tree, fell to the ground with a thud, and cut her arm quite badly. I judged it completely wrong. I felt that pang of guilt. But then I was quickly able to forgive myself. I was trying, I thought. It's okay, she's okay. Then I apologized to her. I explained to her that part of parenting is learning when to help and when to let her figure it out. I told her no one tells you how to parent, that I got this one wrong, and I was sorry. I told her I was proud of her for trying and I was sorry she hurt her arm.

We hugged and it was a beautiful moment of connection. I think I taught her some valuable lessons in that moment; we all mess up, we take responsibility when we do, and there's nothing wrong with messing up. That last one is important. Children will blame themselves over their parents, because it's safer to make themselves wrong than their parent, who is their world.

Someone once saw me do this with my eldest daughter. He looked like he was going to say something, and my ego perked up, wanting a 'Wow, that was impressive' type of comment. Instead (because life is imperfect) he said to me, 'What are you doing? You can't say to your child that you made a mistake. They need to know who's in charge.' It's so fascinating that we've been taught that to be in charge means to be impenetrable, never admitting a mistake, or taking responsibility, when we all know that the best leaders do the opposite. And as parents, we *are* leaders.

Motherkind Toolkit: How to repair

1. Get on your own side first: 'I did something I'm not proud of, and that's okay. I'm allowed to be imperfect.'
2. Go back to the moment of disconnect: 'I've been thinking about when I told you to be quiet a little too loudly the other day.'
3. Acknowledge the impact: 'I guess that might have felt scary to you.'
4. Say what you'll do next time: 'I'm working on how to stay calmer, so I'll shout less next time.'

Motherkind Community: Kelly's story

My client, Kelly, found the early months of parenting challenging yet fulfilling. Although exhaustion and loneliness crept in during her maternity leave, overall, she was enjoying being a mum. It wasn't until she returned to work that things began to change. She was initially excited, but then a shift began inside her. Imposter syndrome hit her hard at work, and balancing her job over four days a week became increasingly difficult. She felt like a complete failure, and her mind was constantly torn between work and home, and all the things she should be or should be doing. The result was that her inner critic grew louder, and she was consumed with an intense anger she couldn't explain.

'Behind closed doors, I would explode over the smallest things, and I was highly triggered by my son. I had become an irritable, impatient, shouty mum – everything I had experienced growing up and swore I would never be. Yet here I was, repeating the same pattern.'

Guilt and shame overwhelmed Kelly, and she despised the person she had become. She felt that she wasn't good enough for anyone, especially her son and husband. At her lowest point, she even contemplated not being here anymore. From the outside, no one had any idea anything was wrong, including her closest friends. She wore a permanent smile and masked everything she was feeling. When we began working together, Kelly began to unpack her limiting beliefs of not being good enough.

'I slowly released the pressure I was putting on myself to be the perfect parent. I learned valuable tools and strategies to let go of control, quiet my inner critic, and develop healthier coping strategies. One of the greatest lessons I learned was that love is in the repair. If I shouted at my son or acted in a way that went against my values, it was okay to step away and then apologize to him, explaining my feelings without condoning my outbursts. It really helped me to improve my connection with him, and my guilt started to dissolve. No day is perfect, that's not life, but I now have unwavering confidence that I am a good mum, doing my best for my children. Because I can hold my own feelings, I am so much more comfortable and equipped to hold theirs.'

Nothing went to plan, and it was beautiful

The best thing about freeing ourselves from the binds of perfectionism is that we have more energy, more joy, and more fun to share with our children. It's ironic that in striving to make things perfect for them, we risk missing out on the actual perfect little moments.

Without doubt, the best moments I've had in motherhood so far have been when I've let go of perfectionism. It's when I've jumped in the paddling pool at my girls' begging. When I've let them stay up late to have a bedroom disco. When I've given cereal for three meals in a row and we've all laughed about it. It's when I've shaken off the armour of the rules and the 'shoulds' and the self-judgement. It's when I've allowed us all to be deeply imperfect, messy humans.

One of my favourite memories from my childhood is sleeping under the stars on a sun lounger. My parents had lost the keys to the holiday apartment we were renting and the agent couldn't get replacements to us until the following day. I can still remember the excitement as my parents told us we'd be sleeping outside. I was thrilled, looking up at the stars, listening to the crickets, wrapped up in a slightly damp beach towel. I felt so happy. I've since spoken to my mum about that night, and she told me she spent the whole night worrying about us, beating herself up for messing up. All the while creating one of my favourite memories. If only we could give ourselves a break.

The more we try to make something perfect, the harder it is when things don't go to plan. Lower expectations usually equal a happier outcome. That is why unplanned things are often the best, because there are no prior expectations. When something is spontaneous or unplanned it frees us up to enjoy whatever happens, without the weight of expectation for how it 'should' be.

I once supported a mother who felt utterly overwhelmed. She was always rushing to the next thing, her mind continually scanning forward to what she had to do and be in the next moment. She was rarely relaxed and tried to control everything around her. She was scattered, stressed, and always had an ache or pain. She was holding on – tight. We'd been working together for a while when she decided that she wanted to get up ten minutes before her children to have a hot coffee in peace before the chaos ensued. One morning she was creeping down the stairs when she heard a little, sleepy voice shout 'Mummy.' In that moment she realized she had a choice: go down her old path of frustration and annoyance that her plan wasn't working out perfectly or make a different choice to let it be imperfect. She chose the latter and went down a new path.

She went into her daughter's room and met her with a smile. They went downstairs together, and she made them both a drink. They cuddled on the sofa and her daughter slipped her little hand into hers. They laughed at how loud the birds were. Tears started streaming down her face as she realized she hadn't felt that connected to her daughter in a long time, or that present. In that moment, it was imperfectly perfect. She took that experience into her day, letting things be, controlling less, letting plans go wrong, and she messaged me that evening to tell me she'd had the best day of motherhood so far. 'Nothing went to plan, and it was beautiful,' she wrote.

Hannah from the Motherkind community told me about a stressful bedtime with her three young boys. 'It was like Whac-A-Mole,' she said. 'All three in the same room trying to get them down.' She thought she'd hit the jackpot when all three were silent. 'Yes!' she thought. 'Dinner and sofa time.' Then through the silence came a little voice. 'Mummy,' said her three-year-old. 'I'm jam, come and lick me.' All four of them howled with laughter. She bottled that moment, and it kept her going all week, remembering the pure joy and craziness of it. Yes, it would take her another twenty minutes to get them down again, but it didn't matter. 'People pay a lot of money for a moment of pure unadulterated joy like that,' she said. 'I'm soaking in every single second of it.'

How to let go a little

Sometimes perfectionism can be having to have things a certain way. It can mean writing endless lists for your partner or child carer when you leave for a few hours. It might be not letting anyone else help you around the house, because they don't do it 'right'. Sometimes perfectionism is a lot like control. Clinical psychologist Dr Emma Svanberg told me, 'When we feel that something is stressful or overwhelming, we try to bring it under our control. We try to make it neater, more predictable – a coping strategy that might leave us feeling calmer for a short period of time.'

Motherkind Community: Beth's story

'One of my biggest fears is my children growing up and realizing I let control and fear steal the moments of joy that could have been sprinkled throughout our journey. When I had my first daughter, I found life with a baby really tough. I didn't find loving her hard. I found everything that came with having a baby tough. I felt like it didn't come naturally to me. I worried a lot and felt anxious and very unsure of myself. I found the days long and the nights even longer. The loss of control that came with a newborn stressed me out. The constant changing nature of everything scared me. The intensity overwhelmed me and realizing my life had changed made me feel sad. It's hard being a mum in the modern world.

I now see that my way of coping, my defence against all this change, and my way of managing my matrescence, was control. Looking back to those early days of my matrescence, I used control to navigate through my days, and it saved me. I became as efficient as I could. I'd organize everything with meticulous planning, endless lists, and many schedules, as it made me feel safer and more in control. I felt like if I had a handle on things, I could cope. In reality I was desperately trying to control something that wasn't meant to be controlled. But it was the only way I knew how to get through those early days. As the years went on and my daughter grew up, I eased into the transitions of matrescence and life became easier. But I had set up a rigorous routine that we had adopted as a way of life and it kind of worked. Until one day I realized, we had no room for joy. Control had sucked all the joy out of our days.

At times I'd shudder if she wanted to jump in the paddling pool because it would mean washing her hair, and Tuesday wasn't a hair-washing night. Or if my husband suggested we ate out, but it was a Thursday and I'd planned to cook sausages. When I started to unpick what had happened, I realized that the control I exerted in those early days had followed me through into a phase of our lives where it was no longer needed. I set upon the task of shedding the control, letting go of the ties I had placed around my life to keep everyone safe. When I did this things started to feel lighter. We stayed up late, jumped in the paddling pool and ate waffles for tea.'

Controlling and micromanaging are exhausting, but they can also help us to feel safe when so much around us feels out of our control. So sometimes control helps us, sometimes it hinders us. The important thing is for you to have awareness of what controlling costs you and how it serves *you*.

Motherkind Toolkit: What control costs you

Using the example below, make a list of areas of your life where controlling both costs you and serves you.

What does controlling cost me?	How does controlling serve me?
I would have more time to myself if I allowed others to help me more	A sense of safety and ease that I have done things the way I want them done

Ask yourself:
- What do you notice?
- Are there areas where you can let go of control a little?

Motherkind Toolkit: Practise letting go

1. Squeeze your hands tightly together to make two fists.
2. Notice how this feels in your body and mind.
3. Gently open your palms and breathe deeply.
4. Notice any shifts in your body and mind.

This is the difference between holding on tightly and letting go. You hopefully noticed how much more relaxed and at ease you felt when you opened your palms. This is a great physical example of how it feels to let go a little.

What if we could accept ourselves as we are right now: acknowledge our struggles, celebrate our wins, and see our lives with more perspective. What if perfection is actually being who and where we are right now? What if it's accepting ourselves just as we are? Perspective is the antidote to perfection. It's hard to beat ourselves up about a seven-year-old falling out of a tree when we imagine our eighty-year-old selves smiling at how hard we were trying, how wonderful we really were.

I read once that each of us has a 1 in 400 trillion chance of being born. Here we are, beating ourselves up about a mistake, panicking about a missed appointment, worrying about being judged, fretting about a ball dropped, complaining about the weather, stressing about whether another mum likes us. When we're miracles, each and every one of us. You're reading this with a heart that beats, on a planet that spins on its axis in the middle of a universe we don't understand. Our bodies produce just the right milk for our babies, breathe without even trying, and grow new humans. What if, even for a split second, we relaxed into the wonder and mystery of it all? What if we realized we're everything and nothing? What if we stop for just a moment and realize how incredible we are? Each of us. All of us. What if we started having our own backs?

If you only have five minutes today ...
- Perfectionism is often misunderstood. It isn't about being perfect, it's about trying to be.
- Perfectionism means you strive for high standards and are never satisfied with what you have done.
- We aren't born perfectionists; we develop these behaviours in childhood to get praise and crave it still in adulthood.
- The root of perfectionism is the belief that we're not good enough.
- We are the first generation to be parenting with social media, which causes endless challenges.
- Freedom from perfectionism is working out what 'good enough' means to you and working on your core beliefs (see Chapter Two).
- We don't need to perfect be parents for our children. For them to develop resilience, we need to be 'good enough'.

- Repair is one of the most important skills we can learn. We all mess up, and learning to apologize and repair strengthens our relationships.
- Control and micromanaging are two characteristics of perfectionism. Both can bring a sense of safety, but block joy and spontaneity.
- We need to realize how incredible we really are and give ourselves a break.

Chapter Five: Your needs matter

'What if a responsible mother is not one who shows her children how to slowly die but how to stay wildly alive until the day she dies? What if the call of motherhood is not to be a martyr but to be a model?'

GLENNON DOYLE, AUTHOR OF *Untamed*

My friend once sent me a message that blew my mind. It said: 'My needs are just as important as everyone else's in this family.' I had to read it a few times to let it really sink in. It's so obvious: there is no hierarchy of needs. Yet I was living my motherhood as if my needs were below everyone else's. I have spoken with thousands of mothers since starting Motherkind and I am yet to find one who has found caring for herself and her needs easy. I want to change that for you.

Four years ago, I slumped on the sofa, stained with milky spills and colouring pens, and put a kid's television show on to entertain my toddler. I felt the energy draining from my body, like a battery draining down, until finally even my toes felt heavy, and I fought to keep my eyes open. 'I've got to get up,' I thought. 'There's so much to do.' The remnants of lunch were still expectantly waiting on the table. Emails needed a response. A podcast needed editing. Wet clothes in the machine needed hanging up to dry (have they passed that threshold where the damp smell is too much?). And there were toys everywhere. I was exhausted.

The truth is, I was four years into motherhood, hosting a podcast about motherhood, running a coaching business supporting mothers, and yet I had no idea how to do motherhood, how to meet my own needs *and* everyone else's. The result was exhaustion. I had to learn the hard way: I can only give when I have something to give from.

Before motherhood it wasn't a skill I ever had to learn. I would regularly feel exhausted, but then I would have a lie-in, or get an early night. I would cancel weekend plans and lie on the (unstained) sofa and binge watch *Sex and the City*. When I felt emotionally exhausted, I would call a friend and talk it through. I would take myself off for a weekend away to replenish. The options to meet my needs pre-motherhood were never simple, but they were much easier.

But once I became a mother, I found it much easier to remind my children to drink water than to drink some myself. I found it easier to facilitate my husband going out for a run than to create the time for me to do the same. I will remind my own mother of the importance of a healthy, balanced diet, and then eat bread for every meal. I lather sunscreen on my children but let myself burn.

But as I've come to learn, the skill of meeting our own needs is vital. Actually, more than vital: it's an act of rebellion in a society that tells us it's selfish to even have needs. It's an act of self-worth to push ourselves further up our own priority list, and it's a gift to our children to have mothers who care about their needs too.

The problem was that when I found myself slumped on the sofa, I didn't know how to break out of my comfort zone of pushing my needs down into the weeds, while tending to everyone else's flowers. When there were competing needs (my children's and husband's), it wasn't a competition at all: mine would always be the ones to go first. And I'm not alone. A 2014 study showed the hierarchy of how mothers prioritize themselves: children, pets, relatives, spouse, then ... us.[34] So, the dog will have rest, two meals a day, snacks, fun, fresh water to drink, and a walk outside, but we might not. And that's not acceptable.

Meeting your needs

A few years ago, I went to a talk given by Dr Gabor Maté. In the question section a mother raised her hand and asked, 'You're one of the leading experts on child development and I understand what you're talking about with attachment, but I'm stressed and busy. So, I want to know, if there's just *one thing* I need to get right, what is it?' There was silence in the cavernous auditorium as we waited for his answer. 'Look after yourself,' he said. Psychotherapist and author of *Raising a Happier Mother* Anna Mathur put it to me like this: 'Imagine a pilot who was exhausted, not looking after herself properly, pushing through night flight after night flight, and refused help from a co-pilot, determined to do it all herself. You wouldn't want to get on that plane, would you? It wouldn't be safe.' As mothers, it's our responsibility to meet our needs, especially our most basic ones for sleep, nutrition, and support, so we can keep showing up for our children.

Back when I worked in corporate business, an impressive woman became the managing director. One day we were chatting, and she said something I have never forgotten. 'The most important thing I have to do now is invest in myself. I've never done this level of role before, being responsible for so many people, and I'll burn out and do everyone a disservice if I don't manage my time and energy properly.' If that new role was motherhood, the opposite would be the case: we become leaders to our children and stop caring about ourselves. As Dr Becky, founder of Good Inside, told me, 'We have to change this idea that parenting is about emptying yourself and being selfless. Nobody benefits. Selfless parenting is terrifying for an adult and terrifying for a kid to have a selfless leader.'

Motherkind Moment
It's non-negotiable to look after ourselves in order to look after our children.

When I look back it's not surprising that I find it hard to care for myself, because children learn not what they're told, but what we see. Elaine Halligan, parenting coach and author of *My Child's Different*, told me that '80 per cent of parenting is modelling'. I observed in my own mother, an incredible woman, that she rarely looked after her own needs. I don't think I ever saw my mum sit down during the whole of my childhood. I saw her clean, cook, tidy, manage, support, give, and love deeply – but never prioritize herself. She would make the bed with me still in it and clear the plates away before I'd even finished eating. Of course, my mum didn't want me to learn that my needs aren't important. Or for me to put myself at the bottom of the pile when I became a mother. 'You matter, my darling,' she lovingly told me. But I learned through *observation* that to be a good mother, wife, and woman I needed to put others' needs before my own. So, when I first tried to express my needs in early motherhood, I didn't believe I was worthy enough to value myself.

I want to break the paradigm that motherhood means a demotion of needs. I am raising two daughters, so it feels vital to show them I am worth looking after, that motherhood doesn't need to mean martyrdom and that when you care for yourself too, everyone benefits. These are the messages I want them to internalize and soak up like blotting paper because that will be the ink they might write their own motherhood with one day. I want them to learn that their worth is a given – just like yours is and mine is – they don't have to do or achieve a thing to feel worthy of caring for themselves. And if they build a family with a partner, I want them to have absorbed from me that their needs are equal.

Motherkind Community: Helen's story

'I've learned the main block to showing up as the mother I would like to be is my own depletion. Charging my own battery, modelling self-care, and taking time for the things I love (as difficult as that often is with small children) are truly the greatest gifts I can give my child. This idea that the greatest trait a mother can possess is to be self-sacrificing is not serving us and is definitely not serving our children.'

The martyr-mother expectation

The app Peanut surveyed 3,600 UK mothers in 2023 and found that 94 per cent felt *expected* to put themselves last and self-sacrifice for families, partners, jobs, and other responsibilities.[35] Whenever we have an expectation for how things 'should be', it's our job to challenge it, so where does this come from? 'I had this invisible poisoned root planted beneath me that said, "Good mothers are martyrs,"' author of *Untamed* Glennon Doyle told me on the podcast. Me too, Glennon.

Perhaps this was something you uncovered in the 'should sham' exercise on page 33? In Chapter One we discussed how our expectations, or 'shoulds', in motherhood come from the messages we've absorbed from the world around us. Perhaps the 'needless martyr mother' is a belief you have absorbed?

Motherkind Moment
Your needs don't disappear once you become responsible for others. In fact, your needs grow.

Our needs are like a beach ball that we try to push under water. We can push them down, but they don't go away just because we ignore them. In fact, they explode up to the surface when we least expect it. We've all been there: we've ignored our need for help, for nutritious food, for support, for water. We've allowed an annoyance with our partner to build, ignored our need for time alone, and then boom: an explosion. The explosion might be screaming at your partner, snapping at the kids, tutting at the slow person in the supermarket queue, or crying on the bathroom floor.

Asking yourself, 'What do I need?' is a really simple question, but one that the thousands of mothers I've spoken to rarely ask themselves. And I get why: we're so focused on everyone else that we might have totally lost our connection with what we need. Emma Reed Turrell, author of *Please Yourself*, told me, 'If you spend more time occupying the feelings and needs of other people than you do occupying your own feelings and needs, you might start to notice you're losing your identity and we don't quite know what we want anymore.' If we're constantly occupied with the needs of others, it's hard to come up for air and ask ourselves, 'What do I need?'

> **Motherkind Moment**
> One of the simplest, most powerful questions you can ask yourself is: 'What do I need?'

A few years ago, I was asked to speak to a group of mothers about my work. I asked them to think about the most powerful question we can ask ourselves: 'What do I need?' I could see tears rolling down cheeks, tiger stripes of make-up slowly emerging, and the feeling in that moment was electric. I wish all of you could have been there. 'That's the first time I've asked myself that question in three years since my son was born,' said one woman. 'I need a rest,' said another. 'I need to slow down.' 'I need to give myself a break.' One woman said it better than I could have: 'My little girl needs me to look after myself better.'

Motherkind Community: Clare's story

When I first met Motherkind client Clare, she was exhausted, isolated, and constantly on edge, expecting an emergency or tragedy. She was also having intrusive thoughts about her baby being injured.

> 'I was running around trying to make everyone else happy. I was tuned into others' needs and anticipating what I thought they needed. When I first heard that I was not responsible for other people's feelings and it wasn't my job to make other people happy, I didn't understand. I uncovered that I was terrified of letting someone down or having someone be disappointed in me.'

Clare was a people-pleaser, just as I was for most of my life. Every morning she would place her husband's vitamins into his hands before he'd even had the chance to get them himself. She had enough to deal with looking after herself and her child, but it took a while for her to begin to believe that it wasn't her job to jump in and take care of others, especially when she hadn't been asked. Clare found that there were endless activities, tasks, and emotional loads she had taken on for others. The turning point was when she began to consider what her life would look like if she put some of them down and focused on what she needed as well.

> 'I needed to flip how I saw the world in order to heal. I felt uncomfortable. It seemed selfish to start focusing on myself, but I felt desperate, so it was worth trying. I had seen the women in my family be martyrs, and I never saw my mother or grandmother prioritize themselves. The unspoken rule was that mothers should not have needs or wants, and they should

also be perfect while they're at it. The trick was to take it slow and keep it simple. It was painful, but I took small, consistent steps to prioritise myself and rewire my brain. Years later, I still frequently pause and ask myself, "What do I need here? What serves me and my wellness?"'

One for me, one for you

Recently my friend was going through a hard time, so I messaged her with a question: 'What do you need?' I could see the three little dots at the top of the screen, telling me that she was typing a reply. I held my phone next to me, waiting to hear how I could help. 'I have no idea,' came the reply. This is something I hear in my coaching practice all the time. Women know that they're not okay but have no idea what they need to get back on track. It certainly doesn't help that we're bombarded with ideas about what we need by the media. A cold shower! A hot bath! No carbs! More carbs! Wake up earlier! Wake up later! So, I want to start with an incredibly simple way to begin to access your needs.

We are so adept at knowing what our children need. We can tell whether they're hungry, tired, bored, or overwhelmed with just a quick glance. All we need to do is develop that same skill for ourselves. However, it can be hard to work out what you need if you've been giving to everyone else but yourself for a while. And if you don't know what your needs are, I want you to know how normal that is. You're getting to know yourself as a mother who has completely different needs to your pre-motherhood self. But it's going to make a huge difference to your life when you can start giving back to yourself a little more.

It was a typical Saturday. We'd just got home from a long day out. The moment we got in, I made the girls a drink each and sat them on the sofa with their screens. 'They've had such a full-on day,' I thought. 'They need a rest.' Then I realized I needed a rest too. My youngest daughter had just started a new nursery and I thought to myself, 'It takes so much energy, a change in routine and new setting' I'm going to make sure she has a few weekends to rest'. Then I realized I needed exactly the same. My eldest daughter started complaining of tiredness a lot. So, I made changes to her diet and bedtime routine. Then I realized I needed exactly the same. We can leverage our skill of knowing what our children need to our advantage.

Motherkind Moment
Working out our needs isn't a new skill we need to develop; we just need to include ourselves in our care.

Motherkind Musing
As you think about what your children need, ask yourself: 'Do I need the same?'

The win-win model

My husband and I are notoriously competitive with each other. Once a therapist said some magic words to us: 'When one of you wins, you both win. When one loses, you both lose.' It's not an exaggeration to say this simple idea changed our marriage. It also changed my motherhood. When I win, we all win. When I lose, we all lose.

Inherent in the 'it's selfish to care for yourself' message is that our children don't benefit from us meeting our own needs. We are taught that filling up our own cups is mutually exclusive from us filling theirs. We're taught it's a zero-sum game, and that is a lie we need to deconstruct. The truth is, everyone benefits from us having our needs met. It might not feel like it in the moment, when you choose to go for a walk alone rather than taking your children with you, and they whine about it. Or when you can't do bedtime because you want to make it to that HIIT class you've been looking forward to all day. Or when you say you can't help them build a fort out of sofa cushions because you want to finish the chapter of your book. It might not feel you're actually helping them, but you are.

> **Motherkind Moment**
> A mother who meets her own needs is teaching her children that their needs matter too.

It's really confusing to tell our children that they matter, that they are important and worthy, when they don't see us treating ourselves with the same compassion. We tell them that they need to eat well, drink enough water, have fun, play, learn, spend time with their friends, make new ones, try new hobbies. But it's confusing when we tell them one thing, then they see us doing the opposite. Let's change that narrative.

Let's be a model to our children, not a martyr

Needs are not a hierarchy or a moral issue, they are part of being human. 'Leaving loudly' is a corporate phrase that means employees (especially more senior ones) make a big deal of leaving early to show that it's not only acceptable but encouraged. It's the complete opposite to the 'leave your jacket on your chair' culture that was alive and well when I was in big businesses in my twenties. We need a similar pendulum swing in our homes. So, I started meeting my own needs loudly. I tell my family: I am going out tonight because I organize playdates for you, and I need to see my friends too. I am going to rest for a moment while you watch television, because just like you need rest, I need it too. I am going to sit and eat lunch with you, because I need fuel just as much as you. I'm going to lie down in my room for a moment because all this noise is too much for me right now and I don't want to snap at you.

We once had a house full of people, and it was chaotic and loud. I popped my head into the destroyed living room (just to check the pictures were still on the walls), and noticed my eldest daughter wasn't there. 'She's gone upstairs,' the chorus of little voices came back. I popped my head into her calm, quiet bedroom. 'You okay, love?' I said. 'I'm fine,' she replied. 'It was loud downstairs, everyone was screaming, and I didn't like it, so I've come up here for a minute to be alone and feel better, then I'll go back down.' 'Proud of you,' I told her with tears in my eyes. She had the idea and then the permission to meet her needs. I could almost hear the generational chains breaking.

Motherkind Toolkit: Your needs

This tool will help you work out what your needs are, and how you might be able to meet them. I think about needs in the four categories below, and I've included a few examples of each:

Emotional	Physical	Intellectual	Spiritual
Connection	Food and water	Learning	Fun
Intimacy and love	Movement	Challenge	Purpose
Vulnerability	Exercise	Curiosity	Meaning
Joy	Sleep	Focus	Nature

Add as many categories as you like and remove any that don't connect with you. Then think about what your needs for each category are. For example, under connection, you might need to speak to your best friend once a week, or a friend every day. You might need to feel connected to your community or your child in a deeper way. You can use this tool as a simple, high-level check-in of your needs, or you can go much deeper. Be guided by what you need.

Each of you reading this will be in a completely different situation. For some, meeting your needs might be easy once you've given yourself the permission. You might have financial resources, a supportive partner, or family nearby. You might have children who don't have additional needs. But for others that won't be the case at all. I could never attempt to work through all the barriers that exist to mothers having their needs met, because sadly the list would probably fill a whole book in itself. Also, my own biases would mean I risk missing many, and the barriers change all the time.

Minimum viable needs

I wish from the bottom of my heart that there was more support, resources, structures, and systems to support mothers. While this is improving, it's going to take time. So, what I can offer you right now is a concept I call 'minimum viable needs'. In the business start-up world, there's a concept called minimum viable product. The idea of this is that you put your product out with just enough features to get your company going. So, by thinking about minimum viable needs, you can begin to meet your needs whatever your circumstances.

Minimum viable needs are about knowing what your 'good enough' is. Using sleep as an example, ask yourself, 'What is the minimum amount of sleep I need every night in order to function and how can I make sure I get enough? What creative ways could I come up with to protect this? Who can I ask for help?'

From the Motherkind community:
'I'm a thousand times calmer with my children now because I don't feel so resentful all the time anymore, because I'm no longer suppressing my needs, which I couldn't even admit to myself I had previously.'

When meeting our needs disappoints others

Now we've firmly established that our needs matter, we have to face another hurdle on the track: in order to meet them, we might have to disappoint someone else. The biggest block I face in meeting my needs is my knee-jerk reaction to put others' needs above my own. I still find it so hard to disappoint, upset, or make another person angry, to the point that it is almost intolerable. I have a programme installed in me that tells me it's easier to disappoint myself than someone else, which is classic people-pleasing behaviour.

A couple of years ago I was walking down the stairs with my eyes fixed on the front door. My eldest daughter was screaming, 'Don't go, don't go, I'll miss you.' It was 7.17 p.m., my breathwork class started at 7.30 p.m., and I was determined to go to it. That weekly breathwork class gave me bandwidth for the whole week – I knew that going would help me be a kinder, more fun, more patient mother. But my daughters didn't want me to go. They wanted it to be like most other nights when I'd stroke their heads and sing them out-of-tune Nineties love ballads. I knew that by taking care of my needs, I'd disappoint someone else – in this case, my children. I remember the first time I tried to leave for an evening class, I didn't make it out of the front door; the guilt and the they matter more than you' inner voice were too strong. I hadn't learned then that I can feel the guilt, hear my inner voice, and go anyway. Learning to tolerate others' discomfort just enough to allow you to take care of your own needs is a skill we all need to learn in motherhood.

> **Motherkind Moment**
> Deciding we matter enough to care for our needs usually involves disappointing someone else.

Reshma Saujani, founder of Mums First and author of *Pay Up*, told me about a study in which a group of five-year-old girls and boys were given lemonade with salt added. The boys immediately spat it out. 'Gross,' one said. 'That's disgusting.' But the girls drank the lemonade, said nothing, and each one finished it. When the researchers asked the girls, 'Why didn't you tell us it was bad?' the girls said, 'We didn't want to upset you.' So people pleasing not only starts from a young age, it's gendered. As Reshma told me, 'We raise our girls to be perfect, and our boys to be brave.'

> **Motherkind Moment**
> People pleasing is the desire to please others at a cost to ourselves.

Those little girls decided to make the researchers comfortable by drinking the salty lemonade instead of spitting it out. They pushed down their own needs to please others. How often have we all drunk the metaphorical lemonade, said 'yes' when we meant 'no', uttered the words 'it doesn't matter' when it really does?

One of my clients, Sam, told me about how she was at the dentist once having root canal treatment. The anaesthetic didn't work, but she was too afraid to speak up, so had the procedure without any pain relief. I cried when she told me that. What is happening to our generation of mothers when we would rather go through pain, physical or emotional, than risk making someone else uncomfortable? It's not innate, it's learned. We have learned to push down our own needs to please others. But the good news is, we can unlearn this.

For so many generations society has expected women to be polite, pleasing, and agreeable. Kasia Urbaniak, author of *Unbound: A Woman's Guide to Power*, told me we have to remember that the shift to women's empowerment is still very new in the context of human existence. 'It's only in the last hundred years that many women have gone from being property to owning property,' she said. It's no wonder we find ourselves pleasing and holding back from speaking our needs. The programme we've downloaded is to stay 'nice'. Kasia explained that for so long in our history as women, and as mothers, it wasn't safe for us to speak up and in many places in the world it still isn't. Mothers encouraged their daughters to be 'nice' to stay safe and ensure a man wanted to marry them. Often the only way to survive was to be compliant and pleasing. The height of womanhood was to be selfless. This little diversion into history helps me so much to have compassion for myself, to understand why I find it deeply uncomfortable to meet my own needs and spit out the lemonade.

From the Motherkind community:

'I was exhausted being constantly switched on to everyone else around me, scanning for information that would inform my every move. Exhausted by perfectionist, unrealistic expectations of myself, and others. Exhausted by saying yes to everyone, at the cost of my energy, and even my boy's best interests at times. I would be full of resentment as a result of behaving to ensure what I thought was everyone else's happiness.'

Permission to disappoint

Accepting that we might disappoint others by advocating for our needs is not easy. We need to remind ourselves that just because someone is disappointed about a choice we make, doesn't mean we made the wrong choice.

When I was pregnant with my eldest daughter, I desperately wanted to give birth to her at home. I was so excited about the possibility of welcoming her into the world at home, until I started telling our families about our plans. There was a lot of fear, confusion, and disappointment. I get it, a home birth may seem like an unusual choice. But for the first time in my life, supported by my husband, I was able to stand firm in what felt right for us, and not let the feelings of others sway me. It was the right choice for us AND other people who loved us were upset about it. Both were true. I did go on to have two incredible home births which were life-defining and altering for me. I learned, for the first time in my life, that I can disappoint others to make the right choices for myself. I shudder at the thought of how resentful and angry I would have felt if I had allowed the fears of others to impact the most important experience of my life to date. I'm grateful every single day that I allowed myself to make the right choice for me.

Clinical psychologist Dr Nicole LePera told me, 'As you leave good-girl conditioning and stop pleasing people you'll get push-back from people. The good girl is compliant and needless. This can lead to resentment, chronic pain, anxiety, depression, and various other symptoms that come from having to repress our emotions and ignore our needs, long term. We need to learn that our needs aren't a burden. If we disappoint someone or don't meet their expectations, we believe we're wrong. Guilt consumes us. This is because we live in a co-dependent culture that says we're responsible for other adult's emotions. It's a good sign if people are disappointed with us; it's a natural part of life. The more authentic we are, the more we'll disappoint people. Adults are fully capable of being disappointed.'

I have chipped away at this pattern and now call myself a people pleaser in recovery, to remind myself to keep this in check. I used to think that someone else liking me was more important than me liking myself. I thought it was uncaring to say no. I thought people wouldn't like me if I said no, and that it wasn't okay to put my needs before theirs. The result? Resentment. I felt like a victim a lot of the time, always rushing from one place to the next, doing things I didn't want to do. I had it all upside down and back to front. Saying no *is* loving to the other person. No one wants us to show up out of obligation, silently seething in resentment. After years of practice (and lots of mistakes), I've learned to say no. I've said no to work, to friendships, to holidays, to parties, and everything in between. When I say yes, it's because I truly want to, not out of fear or obligation. It's more loving to you and it's more loving to me. Win-win.

'I choose discomfort over resentment.'

BRENÉ BROWN IN *The Gifts of Imperfection*

Motherkind Moment
The more authentic we are, the more we'll disappoint others.

I could feel the glances of the other women, their eyes on me, my heart beating fast. I'd been invited out to dinner with my new mum friends and the conversation had turned to the controversy of the moment: Prince Harry and Meghan, The Duke and Duchess of Sussex. There was lots of judgement and everyone around the table had the same view, but I didn't agree. I had two choices: keep quiet to keep the peace, or take a risk and speak up. I chose to speak up. 'I don't agree,' I said, and with a wobbly voice I shared my opposing view on the topic. It felt awkward, and I wasn't liked for disagreeing, but it felt important to my growth. The following day my eldest daughter came home from school and told me how a group of children had been saying mean things to a boy in her class. 'What did you do?' I asked. 'I spoke up, Mummy,' she said. 'Like you say, I was brave and asked them to be kind.' You have the right to make choices that feel right for you. You have the right to express yourself authentically and truthfully. Your feelings matter, your needs matter, you matter.

From the Motherkind community:
'Motherkind has made me care less about what people think of me, made me not care anymore about being a good girl (which broke the habit of a lifetime), and made me realize validation comes from within and not from others' views and material things external to me.'

Motherkind Moment
Emotional maturity is being able to do what feels right for you and accepting how others may feel about that.

Where does this pleasing come from?

Emma Reed Turrell, author of *Please Yourself*, explained that our tendency to put others' needs over our own often develops in childhood. As children, we learn to push our needs down to please those around us. We were probably praised for being 'good' and 'easy'. As discussed in Chapter Two, children change themselves to fit in, because they can't change what is happening around them. Emma told me about the following ways we can become people-pleasers.

1. *We learned that our emotions didn't matter*

Were you told to 'stop being silly' when you cried? That 'good girls don't shout' when you expressed your emotions? To 'get up and stop whingeing' when you fell over? Or 'don't say anything if you don't have something nice to say'? Then you might have got the message that your feelings upset other people, so you learned to repress them. Essentially, we might have been taught that how others feel is more important than how we feel.

2. *We were told to 'be nice'*

We might have grown up with the message that happy is good, and other emotions are bad. We learned that being 'nice' is more important than being real, which is why we say we're fine when we're not. We then have to unlearn this as adults and learn that we can express our real needs and still be loved.

3. *We tried to be 'easy'*

This particularly applies if a parent or caregiver was struggling with stress, or someone in our family was unwell or had additional needs. We learned to be 'easy' so as not to add to the burden. 'They use up all the oxygen,' Emma said. 'You might have made yourself small, pushed down your needs, wants, or feelings far, far down and got on with trying to be easy.'

Understanding where this people-pleasing pattern might have come from is the first step in changing the pattern. Sadly, there isn't a magic chip that switches in our brain when we turn eighteen that allows us, as adults, to advocate for our needs. Instead, we keep repeating this pattern until we pause, take a look at what's going on, and learn a new way.

Motherkind Musing
- Do you relate to any of the patterns above?
- What happened when you expressed a need growing up (try to think in patterns, not one-offs)?
- Did you feel you could confidently ask for what you needed?
- What was the response if you did advocate for your needs?

You can be kind and meet your own needs

Breaking this pattern of pleasing takes time, patience, self-compassion, and maybe some humour along the way too. At every turn there's an opportunity to fall back into forgetting our needs, and saying yes when we mean no. But that's okay.

After the pandemic, we decided to relocate to live by the sea. Planning, prepping, and preparing for the move exhausted me – moving house while running a business and having two young children is a lot. I was running on empty. But sometimes in life you just have to push through, and this was one of those times. By the time we moved into our new house, I was equally elated and exhausted. If I'd asked myself, 'What do I need?' the answer would have come loud and clear: rest and reset. But when we are low on reserves, we are more vulnerable to falling back into unhelpful patterns. So, I didn't ask myself that question. Instead, I kept pushing on through and didn't look after my needs at all. I was now living in an unfamiliar area where I knew no one, and with the school summer holidays looming, I put myself bottom of the pile again. And it cost me: I burned out.

This was a humbling experience. To think I had changed these patterns and then to see myself stuck in them again was really powerful for me. To find myself on the floor, exhausted, and annoyed at myself with nothing left to give my girls reminded me of why I'm so passionate about sharing the Motherkind tools, and how high the cost can be when I don't follow my own advice.

For months I felt guilty at how emotionally unavailable I'd been for my girls when they were at a massive transition point in their lives. But I had to practise what I preach: guilt keeps us stuck, compassion moves us forward. So, I chose to look at myself with compassion. I, too, was going through a massive transition, and at a time of stress, I fell back on my old patterns. I forgot to care about my own needs. And that's okay, I'm only human. I can't expect myself to be perfect, that serves no one. So, I softened, forgave myself, spoke to the girls about it, and learned again how I can help myself in these moments.

I asked expert Emma Reed Turrell how we can change these patterns, and she gave one of the best, simplest answers I've ever heard to a complex puzzle. 'Think about what you want now, your short-term fix. That is probably to avoid conflict, to keep the peace, to make things easy for others, to keep quiet. And then ask yourself, "What do I want most?" What you want most is probably to have authentic relationships, to be true to yourself, to meet your own needs, to value yourself.'

What I want 'now' most of the time is to keep the peace and to avoid any tension or conflict. But what I want 'most' is to be someone who can advocate for my own needs, someone who can risk disappointing others to care for myself. Emma shared that acting on the 'what you want most' is where the reprogramming starts, where we begin to break these habitual patterns. And we're going to dive into that in Chapter Six.

Motherkind Community: Michela's story

'I wish for you to be as kind to yourself as you are to your children, making it a non-negotiable to meet your own needs too. I wish for you to make peace with yourself and the mother you are, knowing that you are doing the best you can with what you've got, in hard times. Because when you as a mother feel well, the rest of the ecosystem of your family benefits too. When you treat yourself with compassion, and your children watch you model this, that changes a whole generation of children who grow up with self-love and self-respect, instead of self-sacrifice and self-criticism.'

If you only have five minutes today ...

- Meeting our needs in motherhood is vital because we can only give when we have something to give from.

- The martyr-mother expectation is the idea that 'good' mothers are expected to put themselves last. This is often the societal messaging we have absorbed.

- When we become mothers, our needs become more important. They don't go away if we try to ignore them; instead, they cause anger, frustration, and exhaustion.

- Asking yourself, 'What do I need?' is simple yet hard because you might not know the answer.

- One way to access your needs is to think about what your children need, because you can often need the same thing. We are typically very skilled at knowing what our children need, so can use that to our advantage.

- There is no hierarchy to needs. All humans have equal needs and when we meet our own needs, everyone benefits.

- It's confusing to children when they see us meeting their needs, but not our own.

- Working out what your needs are is vital because you can only act on what you're aware of.

- 'Minimum viable needs' is a model you can use to meet your needs whatever your circumstances.

- Meeting our own needs can involve disappointing others, which is challenging for those of us who are people pleasers.

- Research shows that people pleasing is gendered and starts at a young age.

- We are allowed to disappoint others in order to please ourselves, and doing that is part of recovery from our 'good girl' conditioning.

- We can change our people-pleasing behaviour by unlearning that our needs don't matter and relearning that we matter.

Chapter Six: Why self-care doesn't work

'I think that most mothers would say that motherhood is the most important, meaningful, rewarding and precious experience of their life, and that it is also the most demanding, stressful, and most draining.'

DR RICK HANSON, PSYCHOLOGIST

When my eldest daughter was a toddler, she cried a lot and I often found my mind wandering off to a point where I would be there in body, but not in mind. I couldn't emotionally connect with her in those moments, and I felt like such a failure. The best way to describe it is feeling spaced out, like a grey fog coming over me. Psychologists call this 'disassociation'. I truly believed that it made me a bad mother. It was only when I started interviewing experts on the nervous system that I understood what was happening: her crying triggered my stress response. I realized I'd always had that response to big emotions, it's just that I'd never noticed before because I'd never been around such constant intense emotion before and I'd never wanted to stay emotionally connected so badly before (or to 'stay in the room' as my therapist calls it).

I made it my mission to learn all I could about how to change this response, so I could be the mother I wanted to be. I wanted to be able to be the 'steady ship in the storm' that so many parenting experts talk about, but I couldn't do that when I was constantly being hijacked by my stress response. Unlike most other situations,

I couldn't just walk away when my baby was screaming. I couldn't change that both my children needed me at the same time, or that both of them ran in opposite directions in the park. So, my question became: if I can't change my stressful surroundings, how can I change my stress response? Psychologist Dr Rick Hanson told me, 'Studies have corroborated what mothers report: being home alone with one or more young children can be very stressful – in fact more stressful than many jobs, as shown by cortisol levels. It's not surprising given the well-known factors of stress: frequent interruptions, emotionally demanding, lack of control, need for multi-tasking, and relentless pace … all landing on a body and mind that is probably sleep-deprived, physiologically drained, and under-nurtured.'

Motherkind Moment
We can't change the stresses of mothering, but we can change how we respond to that stress.

As I write this, it's 7 a.m. and I'm sitting up in bed with my two girls sleeping soundly either side of me. I'm desperate for a sip of water, so I slowly lean over to grab the glass on the bedside table. When replacing it, trying to have the skills of a silent ninja, of course it drops to the floor. The bang makes my heart race. I can feel my face getting hot and anger rising in my body. This is my stress response. I take some deep breaths and I can feel myself coming back to calm (or regulating, as psychologists call it). How many times a day do we deal with a metaphorical (or actual) dropped cup? The stressors in motherhood are constant: crying, whining, screaming, potential danger, throwing, arguing, shouting. Motherhood is essentially a constant assault on our nervous system.

Why we need to understand the stress response

What if I told you that it was totally normal to want to hide in the downstairs bathroom when your children are fighting? Or to shout when you're late and no one will put their shoes on? Or to zone out when you're being asked for the hundredth time where that toy is? That is your stress response; it's automatic and totally normal. There is nothing wrong with you for having these reactions.

Every time we are overwhelmed or overstimulated (which may be most of the time we're with our children), our nervous system responds in one of four ways: flight (wanting to run away), fight (wanting to shout), freeze (wanting to leave your body or quickly becoming overwhelmed), and fawn (wanting to please to make the threat go away). Clinical psychologist Dr Nicole LePera told me, 'The nervous system is like an alarm system in the body.'

When I learned about these reactions and started noticing how often I felt them in my body, it was like I'd been given a new map to understand myself. I noticed how when the girls were climbing on me, I wanted to push them off and run away (flight). How when they'd scream and fight, I'd suddenly feel a rush of rage (fight). How when they'd ask me for the hundredth time for more screen time, I'd give in (fawn). Or how during a particularly intense melt-down, I'd zone out and start thinking about something else entirely (freeze).

> **Motherkind Moment**
> Our four stress responses are fight, flight, freeze, and fawn.

These reactions are totally normal and instinctive, and as self-compassion expert Dr Kristin Neff told me, 'This is our most instinctive way to try and feel safe.' In fact, we share this safety system with all animals and these physical reactions developed to keep us safe in threatening situations (such as being chased by a lion). However, in the modern world these stress responses are triggered all the time by everyday stressors. Understanding your stress responses will free you from feeling any guilt for what is a totally normal reaction.

Motherkind Moment
When my day is stressful, I will be kind to myself for my normal stress response.

Since learning that we all have tendencies to default to certain stress responses (mine are freeze and fawn), I've doubled-up my compassion for myself. I am way more likely not to hold a boundary I've set (fawn) to avoid conflict, or dissociate from the situation entirely (freeze), than I am to shout (fight), or want to leave the room (flight). We also have different levels of stress we can handle before this stress response kicks in (called the 'window of tolerance').

I can never compare myself to a mother who can handle her three children melting down at the same time with ease, when just my three-year-old's tantrums send me over the edge, because we have different nervous systems and different stress responses. Our ability to handle and regulate these stress responses also differs depending on our histories. If you have trauma such as abuse, racism, neglect, addiction, or a lack of emotional support from your childhood, then your nervous system might already have a lower capacity for holding stress. And when we're stressed, we tend to revert to how we handled stress during our childhood.

Dr LePera told me, 'What we will all do when our nervous system is dysregulated ... we'll return to our earliest strategies.' So, if you used to run away and hide in your room a lot as a child, then you might find yourself wanting to do that now too as a parent. It's fascinating to observe your own stress response – to watch yourself react as if watching a play – because over time you'll be able to pause before shouting, or breathe before wanting to run out the door.

Motherkind Musing
- What is your typical stress response? (Think about how you respond to crying, shouting, defiance, things going wrong, being late, or anything that stresses you out.)
- What are the physical and emotional signs you notice?

How to stay calmer in (almost) any situation

When my eldest daughter was just a baby, I started seeing a therapist who specialized in the nervous system. 'I know I have to keep calm when she's screaming, I know about co-regulation, and I need to be her steady ship,' I said. 'But I just can't seem to do it.' My therapist nodded her head knowingly. 'Zoe, your head has all this knowledge, but your body doesn't know that. Your body is really quickly going to stress because it doesn't feel safe, and we need to help you change that. It would be the same if the fire alarms started going off in your house; you wouldn't be able to think straight. And it's the same when our stress response kicks in. When we're stressed, we don't have much choice about how to act, and that's what we need to change.'

I learned that my nervous system was in a state of constant activation and my body was often scanning for a threat, meaning I rarely felt at ease. Essentially, my alarm was often going off and I hadn't learned the code to turn it off. Kimberley Wilson, author of *How to Build a Healthy Brain*, told me: 'Long periods of stress are really not what the brain or the body are adapted for. Your stress response system is adapted to be activated rarely, and acutely, for example when we were back on the savanna and needed to run away. Once you got away, you could come back down from your elevated stress level. What we have now is an environment and a lifestyle of chronic stressors.'

> **Motherkind Moment**
> We have two nervous system responses: alarm and calm. We can learn how to turn off the alarm and move to calm.

Over the next four years I practised and tried everything I could to turn that alarm off: cold showers, breathwork, yoga, walking, humming, singing, dancing, and meditation. I was learning how to switch from my sympathetic (alarm) system to my parasympathetic (calm) system.

Focusing on these ways to calm my system worked and for the first time in my life, I connected with my body and started to feel calmer. I knew it was working when I could stay present when one of my girls was having a meltdown. I could stay with her, I could be her calm presence, and because of something magical called 'mirror neurons', the more I was able to regulate and calm myself, the calmer my girls became. Psychologists call this co-regulation. Emotions are contagious, so the quickest way to help calm our children is to be calm ourselves. So, if we want to be able to help our children quickly move through a tantrum, or help them handle school playground sadness, then we have to learn to calm our own stress response first.

This is why the idea that it's selfish to care for yourself as a mother is insane: taking care of our own needs is literally the least selfish thing we can do. Learning about my stress response has helped me to become a different parent. I'm now a parent who is able to support my girls emotionally when they need it most; a parent who can handle a meltdown without screaming and shouting; a parent who is teaching her girls the life skill of how to handle stressful situations.

Dr LePera told me, 'To create a safe environment begins in the nervous system in your own body. This is why "do as I say, not as I do" doesn't work. We are always attuned to the energies of other people around us, and even if we have someone saying the right things, but their nervous system is in their own stress response and they're telling you to calm down, it doesn't work.'

Motherkind Moment
Learning how to calm our stress response is a gift we give ourselves and our children.

Motherkind Toolkit: Breathing exercises
Breathing exercises are one of the quickest and easiest ways to move out of a stress response and return to calm. The moment things start to get stressful at home or work, I stop and do one of these breathing exercises. It works every time. Pausing when everything is going crazy around you can feel counterintuitive, but calming yourself down first really is the best thing you can do.

It's a good idea to practise these exercises when you're feeling good, so that when you need them in a stressful situation, they are easier to remember.

Box breathing

1. Breathe in for a count of four.
2. Hold your breath for a count of four.

3. Breathe out as you count to four.
4. Hold for a count of four.

Straw breath

1. Take a deep breath in, expanding your belly.
2. Breath out for as long as possible with your mouth shaped as if you're drinking from a straw.

When the stresses build up, we burn out

A psychology professor asked her students, 'How heavy is this glass of water I'm holding?' Students shouted out answers ranging from eight ounces to a couple of pounds. She replied, 'The absolute weight of this glass doesn't matter. It all depends on how long I hold it. If I hold it for a minute or two, it's fairly light. If I hold it for an hour straight, its weight might make my arm ache a little. If I hold it for a day straight, my arm will likely cramp up and feel completely numb and paralysed, forcing me to drop the glass to the floor. In each case, the weight of the glass doesn't change, but the longer I hold it, the heavier it feels to me.'

It was when Emily and Amelia Nagoski, authors of *Burnout* (which examines burnout from a female perspective), shared with me their definition that my own experience started to make sense: 'Burnout is when you have cared too much, for too long. It is the emotional exhaustion when you are overwhelmed and exhausted and still feel like you need to be doing more. I don't know a single woman who doesn't resonate with the experience of just, I feel like I've used up everything I have, and I'm still not meeting the standard that I feel like the world is setting for me. I'm overwhelmed and exhausted by everything I have to do. And I still worry that I'm not doing enough.'

Burnout in motherhood has reached an all-time high. Motherly's

2021 State of Motherhood survey showed that 93 per cent of mothers reported feeling burned out[36] – so I want you to know that if you're feeling burned out, then you're not alone.

> **Motherkind Moment**
> Burnout is the emotional response you experience when you are overwhelmed and exhausted and yet still feel like you need to be doing more.

Selina Barker, author of *Burnt Out*, agreed when she told me that 'You feel exhausted, your brain is frazzled, like a fuse has gone and you can barely choose what to have for lunch without feeling overwhelmed. If you're emotionally burned out, you can experience compassion fatigue; you might normally be very caring and loving and now suddenly you don't feel very caring or loving at all. You might even feel resentful and irritated about the people you're having to take care of. The difference between regular tiredness and burnout is that when you're burned out, it comes with the feeling that you really can't cope anymore. And just having a few early nights and a hot bath isn't going to fix it – that barely touches the sides. That's when you know that you're burned out rather than just a bit tired; burnout tends to last a lot longer. So, if you can look back and think, "I don't know the last time I didn't feel this tired," you're probably burned out.'

I was hanging off every word when Emily and Amelia Nagoski told me, 'It's the emotional-exhaustion element of burnout that's most strongly linked to negative impacts on our health, on relationships, and work for women.' My mind flicked back to my first three years of motherhood and all I'd held: multiple miscarriages, family stresses, a career change, my bumpy matrescence, and all without much release. I had just kept going, like we all have to. Sitting in that basement recording studio and for the first time understanding what burnout really was, I found so much compassion for myself. We can't continuously keep on giving and not pay the price. Amelia continued, 'In short, emotions are tunnels. If you go all the way through them, you get to the light at the end. Exhaustion happens when we get stuck in an emotion.'

My best friend Anna laughs at my tendency for exaggeration. 'How many times can something really be life-changing?' she quips as I tell of another seas-parting moment I've had sitting with my microphone. Well, Anna, here's another one. Learning that emotional exhaustion doesn't come from stress, but from not releasing that stress, was life-changing for me.

Motherkind Moment
Emotional exhaustion doesn't come from stress; it comes from not releasing that stress.

Dr Gabor Maté, author of *The Myth of Normal*, calls mothers 'emotional shock absorbers'. And how right he is. We take on so much: our friends' worries, our partner's work stress, our toddler's explosive emotions, our father's illness, all while worrying about climate change and smoothing over yet another family misunderstanding. We absorb others' stresses and emotions like sponges, but if we don't wring the sponge out, we sink. We get burned out. I had always thought that the secret to avoiding burnout was to try to avoid stress, but stress isn't the problem at all; it only becomes a problem when we don't release the stress, or 'complete the stress cycle'.

'A lot of us are taught that if we fix the problem that caused the stress or the emotion, then we will have dealt with the emotion itself,'

Emily Nagoski told me. 'But that's not the case. You can take the stressor away, but you need to deal with the stress.' It's like my kids doing crafts; I can prise the paint off them, but I still need to deal with the pink handprints all over the table. I now think of releasing the stress that builds up during the day like wiping the table. I get myself a metaphorical clean slate, so I can pile more stress on tomorrow.

When we hold our toddler's emotions, we've dealt with the stressor but not the feeling of stress and frustration. When we've gracefully handled a family member judging our parenting methods, we still need to deal with the feelings of anger and disappointment. And when we've felt that seething resentment of watching our partner casually walking out the door to see his or her friends without having to think about childcare, dinner, or who is going to do bath time, we can't push that resentment down when the door closes. We have to deal with the feelings. We have to complete the stress cycle. And this is how we avoid burnout.

How to release stress

How do you release at the end of a stressful day? When I was first asked this question, I looked embarrassingly blank. I thought to myself: 'Does mindlessly scrolling Instagram count? Numbing in front of the television?' It turns out that completing the stress cycle is free, uncomplicated, and it takes barely any time. As Amelia and Emily Nagoski reveal, the best ways to complete the stress cycles are:

- A short burst of physical activity
- Deep breathing
- Positive social interaction
- Hugging until relaxed (usually for about twenty seconds)
- Crying

I discovered that my own favourite way to release the daily stress is dancing. Dancing activates the parasympathetic nervous system (the calm) and signals the brain to calm, relax, and let go. Peter Levine, a world-leading trauma expert, teaches that animals naturally shake in the wild to release stress. Me and the girls now dance along to our favourite songs most days and shake out the stress. We complete the stress cycle.

A note on alcohol

Did you know that rather than helping with stress, alcohol actually causes it? The 'mummy needs wine' culture is so pervasive (and make no mistake, alcohol is strategically marketed to mothers) and drinking among mothers with children under five has increased a massive 323 per cent since 2020 (yes, the pandemic years).[37] Of course, it makes sense that having a drink at the end of a long day and an even longer bedtime feels like a reward, and after that first sip you feel calmer and happier. I'm not suggesting you need to stop if it's working for you, but I do think we need more education about what alcohol does to our system, because we think it helps with stress, but it actually causes it.

Alcohol causes our body to release adrenaline and the stress hormone cortisol, which is why we may wake up feeling anxious the morning after drinking. So, if you are already feeling stressed or anxious, drinking even a couple of glasses is likely making you feel much worse after the initial rush of calm and ease. It also impacts the deepest, most restorative part of your sleep – REM. So even if it feels like you've been asleep for the same amount of time as usual, you'll feel less rested.

I stopped drinking alcohol ten years ago, and I can categorically say it's the best thing I've ever done for almost every area of my life – there's no way I would have been able to create Motherkind if I was still drinking. Drinking in motherhood could be a whole book on its own, there is so much to unpack and understand, but if you want to start exploring your relationship with alcohol, here are some questions to ponder:

Motherkind Musing
- How do my current drinking habits impact my and my family's lives?
- What feelings come up when I think about cutting back?
- What would I like my relationship with alcohol to be like?
- What actions could I take to explore this further?

A note on sleep

I'm not going to tell you about the importance of sleep. I actually find it hard to read those articles. You may not have had a full night's sleep for a long time. We all know that sleep is important, but often how much we get is outside our control. However, in order to give our exhausted brains and bodies some *compassion* and *validation* – so we can forgive ourselves more quickly when we snap, when we're foggy, when we're at the end of our resources by 5 p.m. – it's useful to know the effects of sleep deprivation.

Lack of sleep causes the part of the brain responsible for emotions to become more active, and at the same time the part of the brain responsible for managing our emotions becomes less active. Think about your emotions as a herd of sheep, and your ability to regulate your emotions as the fence around them. Now double the number of sheep and knock half the fence down. Chaos would ensue, right? This is basically what a lack of sleep does to our emotions.

A study in 2020 revealed that, on average, new parents lose 109 minutes of sleep a night in the first year – that's 663 hours of lost sleep, or 16.5 working weeks.[38] And – take a deep breath – this could take up to seven years to recover from.[39] So, it's vital we're gentle with ourselves and find a way to manage our energy.

A note on fun

Someone once asked me, 'What do you do for fun?' For once, I was very, very quiet. The truth was, as a busy mother of two, I had no idea. I think lots of people think that adult fun is about drinking at a party, but that is absolutely not fun for me (see above), nor is going out for a smart dinner. So I knew what wasn't fun, but what was?

Then I realized that what is most fun for me is connecting with groups of people. So, it's no surprise that through a pandemic, a relocation, two miscarriages, and a new baby I was able to continue releasing a new *Motherkind* podcast episode every single week for six years. Because for me, it doesn't feel like work, it feels like fun. I made it my mission to have more fun outside work and through lots of trial and error I realized fun for me is trying something completely new, like cold-water swimming, which I now do regularly (and is amazing for the nervous system). The key is to figure out what is fun for you and let go of any expectation of what you think 'should' be fun. Experiment, try a few things, and notice what feels good. You are worthy of having more fun.

Motherkind Musing:
- What do I do for fun?
- When do I feel happiest and most alive?
- What would I love to do more of?

Why self-care doesn't work (and what does)

If 'self-care' had a publicist, she would definitely be getting a promotion. The self-care industry is now worth £450 billion globally. Marketeers have cleverly branded their wares as a moment of self-care. Buy this face mask for a moment of self-care. Buy this cream, this quartz roller, this fake tan, this candle. I've fallen for it too, bought the cream, the tan, the candle – I felt great for ten minutes (the smell! The packaging!) and then back to my baseline I went, like a bungee, straight back up again, exhausted and strung out.

> **From the Motherkind community:**
> 'It just feels like self-care is another thing I'm failing at. I get that I need to look after myself to be the woman and mother I want to be, but I just don't have the time, and if I'm honest I wouldn't even know what to do.'

In this book, we won't talk about 'self-care' because it's become a phrase synonymous with two things mothers are often very short of: time and money. I think self-care has become shorthand for things we do to our outer-selves, our shells: nails, hair, skin, and homes. And I'm way more interested in supporting your internal world: how are your energy levels? Do you feel calm? Capable?

Perhaps you're thinking, 'So, I'm supposed to do everything my life demands of me AND do self-care too?' I hear you. That's the problem with the version of self-care our generation is being sold: it feels like another thing to do, with yet more pressure to do it 'right'. I teach *energy management,* which is the opposite of that; it's the very thing that enables you to do everything else you need to do. We have a set amount of energy every day, to get everything done we need to, so doesn't it make sense that we should focus on maximizing our energy?

Motherkind Moment

Let's replace self-care with energy management.

A study from 2017 found that the average mother works ninety-eight hours a week, which is equivalent to two and a half full-time jobs. She starts work at 6.23 a.m. and finishes at 8.31 p.m., which is a fourteen-hour day (and this doesn't include night-time wakings). The same study found that the average mother has just over an hour to herself each day.[40]

When your phone runs out of battery, you plug it in without even thinking about it. It's not a moral issue whether your phone is worth charging or not; if we want it to work, we have to charge it. Just like our phone batteries run down every day, the stresses and pressures of motherhood occur daily, so we need to balance the scales with *daily acts* of energy management. Taking care of your energy is your right, not a reward for when you've ticked off everything on your to-do list (which, let's face it, never happens).

Motherkind Moment

Energy management is something we have to do every day, because the stresses of motherhood exist every single day.

Unlike self-care, which can feel like the cherry on top, energy management is the whole cake; it's the 'how' that enables us to keep going day after day. Psychologist Dr Rick Hanson told me, 'The more stressful your world is and the more it's asking of you every day, the more important it is to grow your internal resources, like inner shock absorbers.'

Your unique energy blueprint

We are all different, so we can't ask others how to do this – we must ask ourselves. We need to become detectives of our own selves and every detective has a method; this is mine: energy givers and energy drains. It's deceptively simple, but paying close attention to what gives you energy and drains your energy is like making a deposit in your energy account and making fewer withdrawals; your energy balance increases.

Most people when they feel exhausted or low on energy think about what they should do more of (sleep, nutrition, exercise); my approach is so powerful because it also invites you to think about what you need to do *less*.

My simple, scribbled list up on my office wall has meant I've changed friendships, set more boundaries, said no a lot more, started running, taken action and had hard conversations. It's given me a map to navigate my needs, it's like a CliffsNotes for the book of myself.

The tool is incredibly simple, completely unique to you, and it works. When I started replacing the drains in my life with the givers, it was like replacing a dull, flickering light bulb – suddenly everything felt brighter and clearer.

Motherkind Toolkit: Your givers and drains

Write a list of at least ten givers and ten drains. Here's some prompts to get you started:

Givers
- When do you feel at your best?
- What do you always look forward to?
- What do you resist doing, but then always feel better afterwards?

Drains
- What do you dread?

> **A few extra tips:**
> - Try to think of some givers that don't use up extra time or money (both will be blockers).
> - Think of some givers you can do when you're with your child.
> - Don't get stuck in the 'shoulds' – yes, yoga 'should' be relaxing, but if you really don't like it, find something you do enjoy.

Motherkind Community: Anna's story

My client Anna described herself as a positive go-getter, who was full of compassion and always had a big smile on her face. However, this all changed after the birth of her second child when she found herself in a dark and lonely place. Anna faced several emotional hardships in a short space of time and did what so many of us do: she put on a brave face, pushed on, and cared for everyone around her. When her daughter was two months old, she lost her mother-in-law to cancer. The loss of her mother-in-law brought back the grief for the loss of her own mother five years before. But Anna didn't process these feelings as she believed it was her duty to stay strong for her family.

'How unfortunate that I did not realize I needed to put on my own oxygen mask before helping others, because eventually I broke. There was no particular trigger. I was sitting on the sofa after putting the kids to bed, and it was as if my soul quietly leaked out of my being. I slowly and non-dramatically deflated, feeling like a flattened balloon with absolutely nothing left inside me. Tears rolled down my cheeks, and I sat, unable to move. On the outside, I appeared fine to most people, but on the inside, I was in shattered pieces. My energy level was at rock bottom, and even doing the dishes felt like climbing Mount Everest. I can still picture myself standing hunched over by the sink, barely able to hold onto the dish brush and tears streaming down my face. I felt so incredibly lost and hopeless, not knowing what was wrong or what to do. I am grateful for my husband, who stepped up in his own kind of way so I could collapse after the kids were asleep. And when the kids were awake, I pushed my feelings aside and functioned somewhat in order to feed, bath, and play.'

The following six months were a blur for Anna, with few memories. Although her husband was a pillar of strength, she had never felt so lonely. She didn't feel understood, seen, or heard, and she felt there was no connection with anyone around her. She doubted her marriage, which made her feel even more lost and lonely. Anna started therapy, which opened some doors but did not shift her feelings of being lost and lonely. What changed for Anna was beginning a journey of self-discovery to connect with her inner child and rediscover her authentic self.

'I learned how essential it is to live by my values and learn what gives me energy and what drains me. I learned to prioritize myself every day with a little bit of solitude to connect with my true self through meditation, gratitude, and journalling. I re-learned how essential connection is. I am now Anna two point zero, and I will be forever grateful. I am positive Anna again, viewing and living life through a different filter – a filter of acceptance and gratitude towards others and myself. I have increased my emotional awareness, improved my communication skills, including setting and following through on boundaries, and am aware of how to communicate clearly to enhance my chances of being understood. I have a great morning and evening routine, which includes gratitude journalling and meditation. I schedule regular reflection and recovery opportunities to live according to my values and energy. Do I still hit bumps along the way? Absolutely. But I now have tools to keep me grounded and to help me recover when I slip. Tools that I actively use to keep me aligned to what truly matters to me as a woman, as a mother, and all the other roles we play.'

Why change (even good change) is gradual

This scenario might feel familiar: you realize you're feeling drained and decide that you're going to make changes. You decide that this is the week when you're going to go to bed on time, do less scrolling on your phone, eat better, and exercise more. Then after a day or two the motivation goes, and you find yourself slipping back into old habits. Then you're back to square one but feel even worse because you're beating yourself up for 'failing' yet again.

One of the most common reasons we fail to make the changes we want in our lives is that we try to change too much at once. How many times have you written an optimistic New Year's resolution list: do more exercise, eat better, change careers, move house. Not only are these terrible goals (way too vague), but you'll never be able to do all of them at once. The secret to change is to choose just one thing from your givers or drains list (and ignore the nagging doubt that this won't be enough to make a difference) and create a plan for how you're going to do it.

Motherkind Moment
The secret to making changes is to start really, really small.

In *Atomic Habits*, James Clear describes how changing a plane's direction by just one degree means it will end up at a totally different destination. It's the same with our givers and drains. Making small changes is not only more manageable, but these small changes will all add up over a few weeks and months to make us feel completely diiferent.

My client wanted to get back to exercise after her second baby, and she told me she wanted to go to the gym three times a week. I said, 'How about once a week to start with?' 'That's ridiculous,' she said. 'That won't make any difference.' But I knew from hard-won experience that we set ourselves up to fail when we aim for too much, too fast. Inevitably we'll fall short of our goals and then our inner critic will have a field day: 'Of course you couldn't do it.' 'You' may as well quit now.' By starting at just once a week, my client taught herself she could keep a promise to herself, and she taught herself she was trustworthy. Over a few months once a week turned to three times a week. Small change, big impact.

> **Motherkind Toolkit: The 1 per cent change**
> Look at your givers and drains list. Choose just one and think about a 1 per cent change you could make today.

I decided a 1 per cent change I wanted to make was drinking a big glass of water before my beloved cup of tea in the morning. I set myself a target to do it for thirty days to see if I felt any different. I noticed the resistance my brain threw at me at the start: 'This is stupid. You don't really need to do this. It won't make any difference.' But I did it anyway. It definitely helped me feel more energetic, so I kept it as a permanent feature of my breakfast-time routine.

Five ways to make healthy habits stick:

1. Expect resistance but do it anyway

Your brain isn't actually that interested in how happy, or energized, or fulfilled you feel. Your brain is only interested in one thing: your safety. And safety means predictability. So, the moment you try to do something different, your brain will resist, because it's a new behaviour, a break from the usual pattern. This is why when you start to implement new habits your mind will tell you, 'It's too hard,' or, 'It's pointless.'

Have you ever rearranged a room but found that your brain still expected to find things in their old places? This is what psychologists call neural pathways in action. We create pathways in our brain and then, to save energy, we don't consciously think about it again, we just automatically go to the place where we expect something to be. Understanding this is the key to being able to make habits stick – we have to create new neural pathways by getting over the initial resistance and continually doing the new action.

2. Don't rely on motivation

Dr Rangan Chatterjee, author of *Happy Mind, Happy Life*, told me, 'If you think motivation is going to be enough to keep you consistent with your changes, you are setting yourself up for failure.' We all know that motivation doesn't last. You might finish this chapter, jot down your givers and drains, and tomorrow do a small action from each column. But the following day it might be harder and by day three you may have given up or forgotten about it all together. And this is perfectly normal, because motivation decreases over time.

How often have we said, 'I'll do that when things are a bit calmer'? Well, things rarely become calmer. The key to something actually happening, like that walk, or coffee with a friend, is to schedule it in. Put it in your diary like you would a work meeting or doctor's appointment. And stick to it.

3. Make it a habit

Research shows the easiest way to make a change stick is to make it a habit. The change then becomes something your brain automatically reminds you to do. The most effective way to make something a habit is to link it to something you already do. So, if you want to make completing the stress cycle one of your actions (e.g. make dancing a habit), then start doing it when you're brushing your teeth. This is called habit stacking, and it's much easier to link a new action to something you're already doing.

4. Watch out for perfectionism

As discussed in Chapter Four, perfection leads to all-or-nothing thinking. So, if you forget about your givers and drains for a few weeks, perfectionism might tell you not to bother, it's too late. But if we focus on growth mindset and progress over perfectionism, then we reframe this to: 'It's so great I've remembered about that, I'm going to put a 1 per cent action in place today.'

5. Track your cycle

Your menstrual cycle has a massive impact on your mood, concentration, and energy levels. If you're working on your energy management, it's also a great idea to start tracking your cycle so you can learn when you're feeling low or high energy. The best time to make changes to your habits is in the follicular phase, in the middle of your cycle (approximately days one to fourteen, but all cycles are different) when you feel happier and more energized.

If you only have five minutes today …

- Learning how to manage our energy is vital because motherhood is the equivalent of working two and a half full-time jobs.
- Our natural responses to stress are fight, flight, freeze, or fawn.
- Everyone has a different window of tolerance (how much stress we can handle).
- Learning about your stress response by observing how you react in a stressful situation will give you compassion and enable you to pause before you react.

- Everyone is different in how we need to manage our energy in motherhood: working out your energy givers and drains is key.
- The best way to make changes in your life is to start small with one thing at a time.
- Burnout is emotional exhaustion, which is holding on to too much emotion for too long, and it's at an all-time high among mothers.
- Mothers tend to be the emotional shock absorbers of the family, and we pay the price.
- Stress isn't the problem, not releasing the stress is.
- The key to avoiding burnout is to complete the stress cycle.
- The best way to release stress is a short burst of physical activity.

Chapter Seven: Your feelings matter

'I thought I was supposed to feel happy. I didn't know I was supposed to feel everything.'

GLENNON DOYLE, AUTHOR OF *Untamed*

I wish someone had told me when I was blissfully thinking motherhood would be all giggles and joy that in reality children are balls of emotion wrapped up as mini humans. My children's feelings came crashing into my world like a wrecking ball. I have never experienced more anger, sadness, frustration, tears, shouting, joy, excitement, and happiness in my life than in motherhood (both theirs and mine). The hardest part of mothering for me hasn't been the exhaustion, the identity shifts, or the mental load. It's been learning to regulate *my own emotions*, so I can respond to theirs.

I wanted to believe that my emotions didn't matter, and that I could raise emotionally healthy children without worrying about my ability to process my own feelings. That I could support the mental wellbeing of my girls by just saying the right things and reading them the right books. I didn't have time to worry about how I felt, I was too busy trying to spin all the plates, and honestly, 'feel my feelings' wasn't one of them.

I've now had the privilege of interviewing over fifty leading experts on emotional health and, much to my frustration, every single one said the same thing: I had to learn how to understand my own emotional world if I was going to help my children with theirs. Raising emotionally healthy children is the challenge of our generation. Child therapist and author of *No Such Thing as Naughty* Kate Silverton told me, 'The biggest thing we can do for our children is to help them regulate their emotions.' We're in a devastating mental health crisis among young people, and expert after expert has told me that emotional health is the *foundation* for good mental health. Psychotherapist Philippa Perry told me that this is the 'most important' skill a parent can learn.

> **Motherkind Moment**
> We can't teach what we don't know, so the first step in raising emotionally healthy children is to develop our own emotional skills.

But what if we weren't taught emotional skills? Many of us weren't taught how to process our feelings so they didn't overcome us, or how feelings can help guide us. Many of us may have even been taught to fear our feelings. Our caregivers may not have wanted to see us upset or angry, so we didn't learn how to handle these trickier emotions. Instead, we learned to push them down. At school, we were taught algebra, but how to manage this vital part of life was missed off the curriculum. Mo Gawdat, author of *Solve for Happy*, told me, 'I think one of the biggest challenges we have in the modern world is they told us, "Don't bring your emotions to school, don't bring them to work," and so what we learned as a result was to hide them.' So, if we're going to break this cycle, we have to learn how to handle all emotions and fill in any emotional skill gaps we might have. Feelings are like maths: you don't just know it; someone has to teach you.

Dr Soph Mort, psychologist and author of *A Manual for Being Human*, told me, 'We are not raised to understand ourselves, we're not taught to understand emotions. Instead, we're raised to fear them, and to experience shame when any kind of distress arises. Rather than being taught simple and effective coping strategies, we're normally taught how to put a brave face on, told to be good, to snap out of it, or that's no big deal. We hide how we truly feel even from ourselves. This means we're totally ill-equipped to manage the stresses of life, and what it means to live inside our emotion-filled bodies.'

It's perfectly normal to have no idea how to feel your feelings or stop them from overwhelming you; after all, many of us weren't taught how to do this. Even Dr Shefali, who has been described as the leading parenting expert of our generation, told me, 'Having my daughter made me realize how underprepared I was emotionally.' And like Dr Shefali, I too realized how much learning I had to do. I'd like to share with you what I've learned.

Motherkind Moment
It's almost impossible to support a child's feelings until you can support your own feelings.

Feeling it all, even the uncomfortable

First, I had to understand that emotional avoidance is not the same as emotional health. Author of *It's Them, Not You* Josh Connolly told me, 'What we need to do is understand that positive mental and emotional health is the ability to feel my range of emotions and know that that's what makes me human.' For as long as I can remember, I've struggled with my emotions. My strategy was to deny them or pretend I was feeling something else. For years when I cried, my inner voice would say, 'You have nothing to cry about,' or 'Pull yourself together.'

For most of my life my one and only goal with my feelings was to feel good. I wanted to be happy, so I just ignored all other feelings, usually by turning on the television, picking up my phone, and staying busy. The result was that it would all become too much, and I would explode, like a pot boiling over. I call it my 'ignore and explode' strategy, and it wasn't pretty. Sometimes I would explode outwards, screaming at my husband, but mostly I would explode inwards. I would turn the anger back on myself telling myself I 'should' be better, that I was a failure, that I wasn't good enough for my girls. Resentment and anger would build up inside me and I had no idea what to do about it.

I didn't know what to do with my perfectly normal feelings of sadness, grief, confusion, or anger, so I repressed them until I was so exhausted I couldn't get out of bed. I had to learn that feelings need to be felt – the word 'emotion' comes from the Latin *emovere*, which means 'to move out'.

I had no idea that to be human is to feel the full range of emotions. I now know that ignoring uncomfortable feelings doesn't make them go away; it makes them come back stronger, like a weed digging in its roots. Kimberley Wilson, author of *How to Build a Healthy Brain*, told me, 'Emotions don't just go away because you don't like them. They're very persistent messengers, they will keep coming around and putting that note through your door saying, "We missed you, but we'll be back tomorrow," and chances are, they will come out as a physical symptom.' Research proves that suppressing our emotions is bad for our health and affects our immune system, making us more susceptible to picking up our kid's colds or even more serious illnesses.[41]

Dr Julie Smith explains in her book *Why Has Nobody Told Me This Before?* that emotions are like waves in the sea – it's much easier to allow them to wash over you than try to fight and resist them. I had no idea that, paradoxically, it was being able to accept all my feelings that would make me feel better. And psychotherapist Philippa Perry told me, 'Think about this: when do you need to shout loudest? It's when you are not heard. Feelings need to be heard.'

Motherkind Moment
Feelings need to be felt. The hardest thing about feelings isn't feeling them, it's trying not to.

Kimberley Wilson told me about a clinical trial that proves this: 'Researchers took two groups of people and asked them to put their hands into ice-cold water. The first group was allowed to express the pain of the cold – they shouted and swore – but the second group was told to stay silent and not show any signs of distress. What do you think happened? Who lasted the longest? The people who were able to express their distress were able to keep their hands in longer. They had better resilience, because the other group were using a huge amount of their energy and their emotional reserve trying to suppress the feeling.'

So, we might have got the idea that emotional resilience is about not showing our feelings, but actually the opposite is true.

But I just want to be happy

In trying to push away our 'bad' feelings, we also deny the 'good' ones. Feelings are a package deal, not a pick and mix. You can't choose happiness, joy, and excitement and ignore sadness, anger, and disappointment. When you turn down the volume on some, you turn the volume down on them all. It's like when you're listening to the radio in the car and you've set the volume level, every song plays at that level. If you want to feel more of the 'good', you must be willing to feel more of the 'bad' too.

Glennon Doyle, author of *Untamed*, told me that, 'We just worship happiness and gratitude, we don't teach people how to also have hard feelings. And so, when I started having those hard feelings, I thought there was something wrong with me.' For a while I thought I just wanted my children to be happy. Of course I did; we all just want to be happy, right? But then I realized that by wishing that, I was falling back into my thwarted 'ignore and deny' strategy. Happiness is a fleeting emotion just like anger and sadness; it comes and goes. No one is happy all the time, and to suggest that is possible is denying our humanness. When we focus only on trying to be happy, we lose our ability to handle the difficult things. If I just wanted my girls to be happy, I'd give them an ice cream every time they asked or let them stay at home when they didn't want to go to school. But they'd miss developing one of life's most vital skills: resilience. So, it's no longer something I aim for. Now I just want my girls to accept their full selves. Author of *I Am Not Your Baby Mother* Candice Brathwaite told me, 'If I'd have learned when I was younger how to process feelings, a lot would have been different for me.'

Under-feeling, overthinking

Our emotions give us incredible information about ourselves, our needs, and our desires. When we can't access them or decide it's too hard to, we tend to overthink. And when we under-feel, we overthink. It was mind-blowing to me that when I started crying more, accepting my anger, and trusting my happiness, I noticed I was overthinking less.

I once had a client who struggled with connecting to her feelings and spent months researching school options for her children. She was going round and round in circles, making lists, interviewing other parents, making multiple visits. 'How do you feel about the different schools?' I asked her. She looked blank. 'I hadn't thought to ask myself that,' she said. I coached her through connecting to her feelings and giving herself more space to notice how she felt in her body when thinking about each option. I asked her which school made her feel calmer and more relaxed. She answered immediately, and knew she'd made her decision. She cried from the relief. Dr Tara Swart, neuroscientist and author of *The Source*, told me, 'If you just think about it in your mind, and it goes round and round, that actually elevates cortisol levels.' Overthinking is stressful, so we have to connect to our feelings in order to minimize this stress. Our emotions are a map of ourselves. If we don't know how to feel them, recognize their messages, and take action, then we make the journey of motherhood a whole lot harder for ourselves.

Motherkind Moment
Our emotions give us incredible information about ourselves, our needs, and our desires.

Learning together

How we respond to our children's feelings tends to mirror how we respond to our own. As psychotherapist Philippa Perry told me, 'If you can't be with your own feelings, to take on someone's so close to you is very, very difficult.' So, it's no surprise that for the first few years of motherhood, my way of dealing with my children's difficult feelings was to try to make them go away as quickly as possible. If they cried, I'd quickly hush them, bounce them, distract them. A tantrum would be met with, 'Don't be silly,' or I'd take the awful advice that ignoring it would make it go away. I did this because that's all I'd ever known for my own feelings. Until I learned a new way, a way for us to learn together.

Getting the NACK of your emotions: Notice, Accept, Choose, and Knowledge

We can't control our emotions, but we can control how we react to them, and it's vital that we teach our children to do the same. Clinical psychologist Dr Nicole LePera defines emotional regulation as 'the ability to feel emotions and cope with them in mature ways'. I have developed a coaching tool, called NACK, which is going to help you do just that.

1. Notice

The first skill in our emotional toolbox is being able to notice what's happening inside us. Noticing and naming our feelings works because, firstly, it gives us the chance to pause before we become overcome by a feeling, and secondly, naming the feeling uses a different part of the brain (the prefrontal cortex), giving us a choice about what we do next. By doing this we're deciding to not let our emotions take over.

The best place to start is to notice how the feeling feels in your body. This doesn't take any time, just a shift in focus. Instead of thinking about it, practise feeling it. Become curious about what it feels like in your body when your toddler has a meltdown, or when you're running late, or when someone ignores your wave in the playground. You might notice your chest tightening just before you're about to lose it at your children. You might notice a knot in your stomach before your first night out with new mum friends. Or a stinging behind your eyes when it just gets too much. Noticing the physical sensations allows you to access your emotional early-warning system. Like parking a car when the beeps get louder as you get closer to another object, you can become your own emotional sensor, so they don't blindside you. This allows you to make a choice about what to do next. Mo Gawdat told me, 'Emotions are very simple to recognize, even if they're very deep inside, because they have physical signatures in your body.'

There's a phrase in mindfulness practice that I love called 'name it to tame it'. When we can name our emotions, we create a small gap of distance from them, which again gives us more of a choice. So, the next step of 'notice' is to put a word to your physical sensations. As you notice your chest tightening and heat rising through your body, before you explode, say to yourself: 'I'm feeling angry.' This simple tool has completely changed my relationship with my emotions and allowed me to be in front of them, instead of at the mercy of them. When coaching groups of mothers I invite each person to say how they are feeling using three words. One client told me this simple little tool helped her feel more connected to her emotional self, and naming the feelings allowed her some distance from them.

It's vital to create pockets in your day to check in with how you're feeling in a similar way to asking yourself 'What do I need?' (see Chapter Five). Dr Rangan Chatterjee, author of *Happy Mind, Happy Life*, told me how important it is to create little moments when we're not doing other things, so we can notice how we're feeling: 'If the first thing you do in the morning is look at your phone, you go straight to social media, emails, then you're literally reacting to whatever the world wants you to look at all day. For many of us that goes on all throughout the day, or throughout the evening, and is still going on when we're in bed in the evening, so we've got no downtime to actually start thinking about our emotions and ask, "How am I feeling?"'

Motherkind Toolkit: Feelings check-in
Take little pockets of your day to ask yourself, 'How am I feeling?'

'Mummy, I'm really angry,' my seven-year-old daughter said one day as her sister stole a block from her tower. She didn't scream, she didn't lash out at her sister; she named how she was feeling. We'd been learning together. She'd heard me say hundreds of times, 'Mummy is feeling angry.' She'd watch me name my feeling, create distance from it, and not explode. We're learning together. This doesn't happen all the time (for either of us), but that it even happens occasionally is good enough for me.

The power of AND

Feelings are not black and white. They are not one thing or the other, this OR that. They are this AND that. I feel angry and grateful. I feel grief and joy. I feel happy and lost. When we allow ourselves to be complex, multidimensional, contradictory emotional beings, it becomes easier.

Motherkind Moment
I can choose not to let my feelings overcome me by naming what I am feeling.

Motherkind Toolkit: Naming your feelings
- Notice what is going on in your body: what physical sensations do you experience as you go through your day?
- Practise naming your feelings out loud in front of your children.
- Practise using 'and' when you feel different feelings.

2. Accept

Every human wants to be seen and understood. It's the best feeling in the world when someone just 'gets' you, when you are heard without someone trying to fix you or change how you feel. Learning not only to notice but also validate feelings changed the emotional landscape of our home. There is such a paradox that in welcoming the emotion and accepting it, it passes more quickly.

> **Motherkind Moment**
> Accepting our feelings makes them pass more quickly.

I first tried this when my eldest daughter was three. She was having a tantrum about me giving her the wrong spoon. Previously I might have said, 'Don't be so silly, it's just a spoon.' Instead I responded with: 'That spoon really matters to you, doesn't it? Do you feel sad about it?' I couldn't believe it when her whining stopped almost immediately, and her little head nodded, tears on her cheek. I had validated how she felt; she felt seen and understood, and it made the feeling pass more quickly. I still didn't change the spoon. All feelings are welcome, all behaviours are not.

Accepting my own emotions was harder, as it seemed illogical that accepting an emotion could make it pass more quickly. It goes against what many of us were modelled growing up: to ignore our feelings, push them to the back of our busy minds, and keep them unspoken.

Imagine you call up a friend and the tears come as you tell her about a really difficult situation with your boss. She either says, 'Don't worry about it, I think you're great,' or 'Wow, that sounds really hard, it makes sense for you to be so upset about that.' Which feels better? Which version of that friend would you feel safer with, or closer to?

> **Motherkind Moment**
> You are not your feelings – they pass and do not define you.

Feeling angry doesn't make you a bad mother. Feeling bored doesn't mean you don't love your children. Feeling frustrated doesn't mean you're not cut out for motherhood. Feeling guilty doesn't mean you are guilty. They are just feelings. And a reason for this is that ninety seconds is all it takes to label an emotion and allow it to dissipate. Dr Jill Bolte Taylor is a Harvard neuroscientist who discovered through neuroimaging that pausing for ninety seconds and labelling what you're feeling (e.g. 'I'm getting angry') reduces your reactivity.[42]

It's not surprising

'I feel so overwhelmed,' I thought, and then, 'What's wrong with me? Why can't I just be on top of it all?' Shaming ourselves for our feelings is like kicking ourselves when we're down. When you're feeling bad, you need your own compassion and kindness more than ever. And this magic phrase will instantly switch your mindset to a kinder one:

- It's not surprising I'm feeling resentful, given that I've done every bedtime alone this week.
- It's not surprising I'm feeling overwhelmed, given all I've got going on.
- It's not surprising I'm feeling sad, given all the change that's been happening recently.
- It's not surprising I feel lonely, given that I haven't spoken to another adult all day.

> **Motherkind Toolkit: Accepting emotions**
> - Practise not judging yourself for your emotion but accepting it by allowing it to move through your body.
> - Practise saying, 'It's not surprising I feel X, given Y.'

3. Choose

I could immediately tell something had happened at school. My daughter's face looked small, like she was trying to hide it from the world, and I could see she'd been crying. 'What happened?' I said. 'Some girls were mean to me, they called me boring and annoying.' I instantly felt the anger flushing my face, my heart beating faster. I was overcome with anger. 'How dare they?' I thought, as my protective lioness roared inside me. But I knew what my daughter needed in that moment wasn't my anger, but for *me to validate and help her calm her feelings.* So, I took three deep breaths to give myself some choice in how I reacted. It worked: I felt calmer as I got down to her level. 'Ouch, sounds tough. How did that feel?' 'Sad' she said, and the tears came – the release when her truth was recognized. 'I'm not surprised, I'd feel sad too if someone said those things to me.' With those words I could see the sadness passing, as it often does with validation. 'What would help you?' 'An ice cream,' she replied. 'Smart girl,' I thought. 'I'm not going to get you an ice cream, but let's go home and have a cuddle.'

As we hugged on the sofa, I could see the sadness had passed. We chatted about mean words, how to visualize protection around you so they don't hurt as much, and how important it is not to believe them. As founder of Hand in Hand Parenting, Patty Wipfler told me, 'Connection is the only thing that's going to get through to your child's brain when it is full of feelings and out-of-control impulses.'

Motherkind Moment

We can't control what happens around us, but we can control our reactions.

When emotions come, we have two choices: we can react in the feeling, or we can respond to it. Both are necessary and welcome, but most of the mothers I've connected with over the years find it much harder to respond, to *choose* what to do with the feeling. Feelings aren't facts and we don't have to act on them, we can learn to respond more and react less.

Motherkind Moment

We can't change our emotions but can choose how we respond to them.

Motherkind Toolkit: Pause

Next time you feel a strong emotion, ask yourself:
- How can I best calm myself in this moment?
- Do I need to act on this feeling right now?
- Is it appropriate to the current situation?
- What would happen if I waited for an hour before acting?

4. Knowledge

Dr Julie Smith, clinical psychologist and author of *Why Has Nobody Told Me This Before?*, told me, 'Emotion is your brain interpreting all of the sensory signals coming from inside your body and from the outside world. So emotion often holds insightful information about what we need.' Interpretation is key, because feelings are not facts, but they do give us information. So, you may *feel* guilty, but that doesn't mean you *are* guilty. This is why knowledge is the next step on your emotional map. When you're in the thick of it, even when you've noticed, accepted, and calmed yourself, it's still difficult to see patterns or look deeper at why you might be feeling a certain way. Having curiosity about your emotional reactions will enable you to examine why you are feeling a certain way and what changes you might want to make as a result.

I wonder why …

I came up with this idea while listening to author Simon Sinek talk on stage in London. I was so far back he was a tiny dot, but the message landed nonetheless: 'start with why'. He was talking about brands, but as is my obsession with our inner emotional lives, I started applying it to how I was feeling and the results were remarkable.

- I wonder why I feel so angry at dinner times?
- I wonder why I feel so frustrated when my toddler keeps asking me to play?
- I wonder why I feel so disappointed when my friend doesn't reply to my message?
- I wonder why I feel so much tension when I leave for work?
- I wonder why I feel so guilty every time I take time for myself?

Asking yourself 'why' takes any self-judgement away, as it's a kindness to ask yourself why you feel the way you do. It tells your subconscious mind that your feelings matter, that you matter, and it will give you so much information about yourself.

One of my clients found herself becoming increasingly frustrated when her son asked her to play with him. She would feel heat rising and her chest tightening as he begged her to play cars. She used the Notice and Accept tools, which allowed her to Choose not to snap and leave the room. But it was when she used the Knowledge tool that things really changed for her. That night she jotted in her journal: 'I wonder why I feel so frustrated when he asks me to play?' She stared at the blank page, feeling so much resistance to the question (a sure sign there is something to uncover). But she was completely committed to becoming the mother she wanted to be, so she started writing anyway, and once she started she couldn't stop. The words poured out onto the page as she connected with her younger self, who never had a parent who played with her. She realized whenever she asked her parents to play, she was told they were too busy, and she made the link between this reaction and the frustration she felt with her son. Sometimes knowledge is all we need. The following month she sent me a picture of her playing happily with her son.

Motherkind Toolkit
When you start to notice patterns in your emotional reactions, ask yourself: 'I wonder why?'

I use the NACK tool most days, and I have seen these steps completely transform my clients' experience of motherhood: they are no longer overcome by emotion or busy trying to avoid it.

A note on crying

Is there anything harder than seeing your children or loved ones cry? My instinct was always to jump in when the girls cried and tell them, 'Don't cry.' But what are we really saying when we tell our children not to cry? It comes from a kind place, of course, but the underlying message is: I'm not okay with your emotions.

Even when we try to offer a different perspective or kind words, we are also trying to stop the crying. When adults cry it can be seen as weak or embarrassing, and through coaching groups of mothers over the years, I've seen how uncomfortable we are with others' tears. I know I'm not alone in my experience of being told to 'stop crying' as a child, or offered advice and solutions the moment the tears started to fall. Through my work, it's been a revelation to discover what an emotionally blocked society we live in (especially in the UK, where I live). It was only when I learned what tears represent that my perspective completely shifted.

Crying is a miraculous process. It's like a safety valve in your body which releases emotion when it bubbles over. Crying activates the parasympathetic nervous system to calm us, and reduces the stress hormone cortisol. In fact, tears have been found to contain cortisol, so by crying we are literally washing the stress away. I learned from clinical psychologist Dr Nicole LePera that crying is your body's way of trying to rebalance itself, which is why we feel much lighter after a good cry. Crying is our body's way of saying, 'I need to release this emotion.' So, when we cut this process short – when we say, 'Don't cry' – we stop the body from processing the emotion it needs to.

> **Motherkind Moment**
> Crying is your body's way of trying to rebalance itself.

Now when my children cry, my perspective is completely different. I know it's their emotional system releasing and rebalancing. Instead of, 'Don't cry,' I now say, 'Keep crying until it passes, I'm here for you.' It's not easy to allow your child to keep crying at the party, or the park, or the playgroup, and your automatic response is probably going to be to try to get them to stop, but by allowing the tears to flow, you're actually helping your child return to calm much more quickly. Sometimes I imagine the stress and pain leaving their bodies in salty streams down their faces.

When I was beginning my journey of connecting to my emotions, I would cry whole rivers of tears. It was as if I had opened the floodgates, and it was scary. 'Will it ever stop?' I thought. Then one day when I was having a big sob a coach I was working with said the most beautiful words to me: 'All these tears are as if the ice is melting around your heart.' And I cried even more because that felt so true. I had pushed my tears down for decades and as I melted into vulnerability, the tears flowed. They did eventually stop, I hadn't opened the floodgates, but I had opened my heart a little more. Now I cry when I need to, and I always feel lighter afterwards.

A note on rage

When my daughter was six months old, I could tell she was overtired. Putting her in her cot wasn't working, so I picked her up and rocked her in my tired arms to try to get her to drop off. I was exhausted from a bad night of broken sleep, and I was desperate to get her down so I could lay down myself. I was trying to stay calm as I rocked her, but I could feel the stress rising in my body as she just wasn't closing her tired little eyes. Then they finally shut, and I could feel the relief in my body. Rest was in reach.

Just as I was creeping out of the room, knowing the quietest route well, I nearly jumped out of my skin at the noise of our little cockapoo barking. Then, inevitably, my daughter woke and started crying. My feelings came hot and fast, rushing through my body as my chest tightened, and in that moment, I had no control. My fight response well and truly activated. I stormed down the stairs screaming the dog's name. It shook me up completely. I had never known rage like that. Who was I? What was wrong with me? Was I a terrible person? I was breathless and shook as I tried to calm myself down enough to go back upstairs and begin the rocking process again.

It scared me and I told no one. I didn't know that what had happened to me was completely normal in motherhood; the pressure and stress had caused me to 'flip my lid'. I had experienced a surge of adrenaline and then my fight response caused me to feel a surge of aggression. As Dr Caroline Boyd, author of *Mindful New Mum*, told me, 'Anger is a normal reaction to stress. It doesn't make you a bad mum, it means that you are human.'

What is going on when we experience anger?

Imagine this scenario: you wake up already tired from a broken night's sleep, your toddler slams the bowl on the floor at breakfast, but you smile and clear it up. 'Doesn't matter, darling,' you hear yourself say. Your older child won't put their shoes on for school, and you're going to be late for your first meeting of the day. Stress tightens your chest, but you manage to take a deep breath, smile, and get everyone in the car. You run to your meeting, hungry and thirsty, willing your brain to switch from parent mode to work mode. You check your email: there's a passive-aggressive email from a colleague. You miss lunch because the meeting runs over. You run to school pick-up and arrive breathless. On seeing you, her safe place, your child explodes with the tears she's held in all day and releases all that pushed-down emotion.

You manage to calm her, but you can feel the toll it takes. You make dinner from scratch, because they've had convenience food every other day that week, while trying to plan the next steps on a big work project. You serve your children dinner with a smile, but inside you're exhausted and thinking about how much work you've still got to do after their bedtime. A loud crash suddenly makes you jump: your toddler has thrown their dinner on the floor. The heat rises in your chest, and you explode. 'What's wrong with you?' you scream. 'Why can't you just eat it?' Your toddler starts to cry, and so does your older child. Overcome by guilt and exhaustion, so do you.

It wasn't your toddler throwing their dinner on the floor that made you angry, it was everything that came before it. Having spoken to hundreds of mums about their anger, I know that this is a common story. It's what I call the 'drip-drip-drip effect.' There is only so much we can take before the pot boils over. Dr Caroline Boyd explained: 'In flipped-lid mode we are beyond thinking logically; our thinking brain has gone offline.'

So, we need to forgive ourselves quickly for our explosions, accept that it's our biology and not a moral failing, and repair if we need to. Dr Boyd told me that 'anger is a signal to an unmet need', which is why it's so important to meet our needs in tiny ways as we go through our days. We need to counter the 'drip drip drip' of stresses with a 'drip drip drip' of meeting our needs.

Fireproofing

The anger has passed, we've forgiven ourselves, and said sorry to our children. We've put the fire out. But if we find ourselves continually having to put fires out, we might need to do some fireproofing. Dr Becky, founder of Good Inside, told me about this vital distinction: 'After you've contained a fire you're back to your baseline,' she explained. 'You have to think about fireproofing your home.'

If anger signals unmet needs and you're experiencing anger often, it might be a good idea to go back to Chapter Five where I show you how to figure out your needs and begin to meet them.

Albert Einstein famously said, 'Insanity is doing the same thing over and over again and expecting different results.' This reminds me that if I want to shout less, lose my temper less often, and be able to process my anger differently, then I must do something different.

When anger is useful

It was anger that first inspired me to set up Motherkind. I felt angry that the content I was being sold as a new mum focused only on my baby. I felt angry that no one was talking about what I now know is matrescence, about the complete and utter metamorphosis that is motherhood. I felt angry that when mothers are offered a solution to the overwhelm, it was alcohol. Anger, when we put reins on it, is a powerful driving force. Psychotherapist and author of *How to Build a Healthy Brain* Kimberley Wilson told me, 'Anger is the emotion of self-esteem. It's a clue to you that you are feeling or seeing injustice.'

It was anger that enabled many of my clients to change jobs, ask for help, do less, and set boundaries. It was anger that drove activist Joeli Brearley to launch Pregnant Then Screwed, an organization that has supported millions of mothers and helped shape government policy. 'I was furious,' Joeli said about being sacked by voicemail when she was four months pregnant. Kimberley Wilson told me, 'Anger is my favourite emotion, because I think it can be hugely powerful and hugely powerful in a really positive way.' Anger is often the first step in beginning to advocate for yourself, to set boundaries, to ask for what you need. Anger, used constructively, is powerful.

Motherkind Musing
- What could my anger be trying to tell me?
- What is in my control to change?
- What do I need to accept?

A note on gratitude

Gratitude holds all my other feelings like a soft blanket – they need each other. If I force only gratitude, I risk falling back to my 'ignore and deny' strategy as I wash toxic positivity over myself in an attempt to deny the hard feelings. We don't want any 'enjoy every moment' trope here. But if I only focus on the hard, I miss the incredible little moments that occur every day. When we bring gratitude to meet the hard feelings, we can see the whole picture.

Never harder, never happier

Gratitude is the skill of being able to notice what is good, even when everything feels bad. Gratitude is becoming a master at noticing the small, seemingly insignificant things, which actually aren't small at all. Gratitude is like putting on a new pair of glasses, and suddenly you can see things more clearly. It's the skill of being able to deeply appreciate what you have and, at the same time, accepting it's never going to be perfect. Appreciating what you have doesn't mean you don't want things to change or that you have to be grateful for the hard things. But it does mean that you sift through, find the good things, and allow them to help you feel good.

It was school pick-up time, I was running late, I had missed an important deadline for the podcast, and I'd forgotten my daughter's snack (which I knew would be met with anger at best, a full-on meltdown at worst). I was feeling overwhelmed, and my head was foggy with stress as I ran to the school. As I stood there waiting, my head still spinning, I saw a beaming smile looking up at me – my little girl thrilled to see me, buzzing with excitement to show me her latest art creation. 'I am so grateful to be here to feel this,' I thought. Then the snack meltdown happened. Grateful AND overwhelmed. We can feel both at the same time.

Whenever I'm feeling low, I think about something I'm grateful for – the smaller the better. The sun shining through my office window; clean, fresh water to drink; hands that enable me to type these words to you. I ask my clients to write at least ten small things a day they are grateful for, with no repeats. Most can't believe how different they feel after just a week. And studies have found that a single act of thoughtful gratitude produces an immediate 10 per cent increase in happiness, and a 35 per cent reduction in depressive symptoms.[43]

While studying economics I learned about diminishing returns, which means the longer you have something the less you appreciate it. This is why gratitude works so well – it stops us ignoring the small things because we've had them a while. The first time I heard the word 'Mummy' it took my breath away. I longed to hear that tiny little voice say those words again and again, and I couldn't hear them enough. Fast forward a few years, and the word 'Mum' hurled at me hundreds of times a day has gone from something I used to adore to something I often zone out. What happened? The longer you have something the less you appreciate it.

So now a couple of times a day when I hear 'Mum', I make an effort to remind myself what a privilege it is to be a mother, and how lucky I am to have these two girls. Just for a moment my mood changes completely.

If you only have five minutes today ...
- It is completely normal to experience a daily rollercoaster of emotions in motherhood.
- Feelings are a part of being human and feeling bad is a part of life – it doesn't mean there's anything wrong.
- We don't always have a choice about how we feel, but we can choose how we respond.

- If we want to help our children with their feelings, we have to learn how to manage our own.
- Many of us weren't taught how to connect to our emotions, process them, or use them as a signal, and so we need to learn.
- Feelings need to be felt, because what we resist, persists.
- Feeling happy all the time is a myth we need to let go of.
- Being disconnected to our feelings means we overthink and look to others for answers, instead of looking within ourselves.
- We can learn how to handle emotions together with our children – they can teach us, and we can teach them.
- NACK is my tool for learning to manage our feelings: Notice, Accept, Choose, and Knowledge
- Crying is our body's way of balancing our emotions and actually helps us reduce stress.
- Anger is normal, we just need to learn how to feel it and process it.
- Gratitude and celebrating the small wins help us to have perspective for the harder feelings.

Chapter Eight: Verdict: Not guilty

'We're the generation that does more for our kids than ever in history yet feels the guiltiest.'

JEN HATMAKER, AUTHOR AND SPEAKER

I'm on holiday as I write these words. It's 40°C, the air is hot and heavy, and I can hear faint squeals followed by splashes in the background as I try to keep myself focused. But I'm not alone. Guilt is sitting next to me wanting to shuffle over and sit on my lap: 'You should be out there playing in the pool too,' it says. 'The girls think your work is more important than them.' Then the final blow: 'You're a bad mother, the other mums are out there playing while you're up here working.' Guilt, shame, comparison. My inner critic has hit the jackpot, three in a row like rotten lemons on the fruit machine. But the difference is that I now know I have a choice.

In the past, I might have slammed my laptop shut, reluctantly and resentfully gone out to play, like a foot soldier to guilt, marching to her unrelenting drum. Or I might have kept working, but with an uneasy feeling of doubt in the pit of my stomach increasing with every passing minute. But not today. I refuse to be dictated to by guilt. So instead, I sit up a little straighter, acknowledge the guilt, then remind myself that I've played all morning, how brilliant it is that my girls can have fun and play with other adults, how safe they are, how lucky I am to have work I can do anywhere, how important my work is to me and our family, and what a great mother I am. And just like that, the guilt has gone. I'm free. I can focus all of my precious energy on writing at least half of this chapter before wrinkly little fingers and sopping hair come through the door, and it's much easier without guilt sitting on my lap.

Before I learned the skills discussed in this chapter, I was often carrying guilt around like a third child sat on my hip. And sadly, my experience is almost universal – a study from BabyCentre revealed that 94 per cent of mothers experience guilt on most days.[44]

Motherkind Moment

We are in a motherhood guilt epidemic, and we need to challenge this.

Before I learned what I'm about to teach you, I felt guilty about almost everything. I felt guilty about how much I struggled with breastfeeding. Guilty about not being able to soothe flowing tears. Guilty that I went back to work too soon. Guilty that my daughters had too much screen time. Guilty that I didn't enjoy every minute. Guilty that we chose the wrong first nursery. Guilty when they had sugar. Guilty when I said no to sugar. Guilty for loving my job so much. Guilty for taking time for myself. Guilty for not taking time for myself. I felt guilty about something big or small on most days. Feeling guilty as a mother is such a universal, ingrained experience, it even has its own name: mum guilt.

Someone once said to me, 'Give birth to the baby, give birth to the guilt.' Well, in this chapter I want to help you completely change your relationship with guilt. You deserve to live your life and mother your children without guilt breaking you every day. I want you to experience the freedom I feel right now of being able to make *a choice* about guilt.

> *'Between stimulus and response there is a space. In that space is our power to choose our response. In our response lies our growth and our freedom.'*
>
> VIKTOR EMIL FRANKL, AUSTRIAN PSYCHIATRIST AND
> HOLOCAUST SURVIVOR

We don't need to hear 'stop feeling guilty'. What we need is to reflect on where our guilt might be coming from and decide what to do about it. Giving ourselves a choice about how we respond to guilt is where our freedom lies. And I want you to feel free. As psychologist Dr Rick Hanson told me, 'What arises when guilt leaves is a bone-deep feeling of worth as a human, and a woman and a mother.'

A new way to look at guilt: the 80:20 rule

The red 'missed delivery' card sat on the kitchen table for weeks. 'I must collect that package,' I said to myself. It was a birthday present thoughtfully sent to me by one of my closest friends. My eldest daughter was very little and even a small bit of life admin felt over-whelming. Weeks turned into months and by the time I eventually made it to the post office, the package had been destroyed. I felt sick in the pit of my stomach: embarrassed and guilty that I allowed my friend's hard-earned money and thoughtful gesture to be wasted. Telling her was mortifying. I apologized profusely, explained how guilty I felt, and promised her I would never let it happen again. My guilt was very welcome, as I had behaved in a way I didn't feel proud of, and which wasn't in line with my values. Luckily, she forgave me.

True guilt is when we have acted out of line with our values, and we feel a pull to do something about it. I felt guilty because I value kindness, and my actions hadn't been kind. It's normally something we can make amends for, just as I did by apologizing to my friend and changing my behaviour going forwards (I have never, ever missed a package from a friend since). Or like when I bashed my youngest daughter's head when getting her into her car seat (who hasn't done that!?). I felt a pang of guilt, said sorry to her, and was extra careful getting her in next time.

This is what I call 'good guilt'. Good guilt, while unpleasant, is useful. From an evolutionary perspective it developed to help us stay part of the tribe, so we felt discomfort when we did something wrong. We need this good guilt as it's a force for positive change in our lives. Psychotherapist and author Julia Samuel MBE once said to me, 'Zoe, it's only psychopaths who never feel any guilt.' This is because we can only feel guilty if we also feel empathy – we can feel how someone might have felt as a result of our actions, and reflect on our own behaviour. Imagine if I'd bashed my daughter's head and made her cry but felt nothing.

Good guilt is actually an amazing signal for the level of empathy and connection we have with our children. So, we need good guilt. It helps us be who we want to be in the world, and to apologize and self-reflect, which are tools we need if we're going to have positive, meaningful, connected relationships with our children.

But I've had thousands of conversations with clients about guilt in motherhood and on average, only 20 per cent of what they attributed to feelings of guilt was *actually* guilt. So where does the other 80 per cent come from?

> **Motherkind Moment**
>
> Good guilt is there to help and guide us; it exists when we act in ways we're not proud of. It's an uncomfortable feeling that helps us reflect and make amends. But most 'mum guilt' isn't good guilt at all, and we need to challenge it.

Guilt is only useful when we can do something about it. If we feel guilty for working or missing something important, but there is nothing we can (or perhaps want to) change, then feeling guilty is a toxic, useless emotion. Let's explore why.

Eighty per cent of the guilt we feel isn't guilt at all. We've been using the word 'guilt' to describe feelings and reactions that are not guilt at all. It's as if we've only had one colour so we've painted our whole selves in it, forgetting about the other shades. Here I'm going to show you the other colours, i.e. what these feelings really are, and what you can do about them. This matters because if we use the wrong label, we use the wrong solution. If we think something is guilt when it isn't, we use the solution of trying to change ourselves when in fact, we haven't done anything wrong.

> **Motherkind Moment**
>
> I deserve to dive deeper into the feelings I have been mislabelling as guilt to free myself from feeling negative about myself.

The T-SIPS: Tension, Standards, Inner critic, Permeating, and Shame

From personal experience, speaking with experts, and working with clients, I've identified five things we mislabel as guilt: Tension, Standards, Inner critic, Permeating, and Shame – or T-SIPS for short.

Tension

There is always going to be tension in motherhood. You can't be in two places at once and whenever you make a decision, there is tension with the choice you didn't make. But this feeling of tension isn't guilt. The moment we can accept that tension is an ever-present companion in motherhood, we'll be able to make peace with it.

Standards

Motherhood studies sociologist Dr Sophie Brock told me, 'Motherhood guilt is so prevalent because we're measuring ourselves against what we have been conditioned to believe is the ideal mother.' When she said that, it made so much sense to me. A 'good' mother makes organic, home-cooked meals every day, so I felt guilty for serving pasta pesto again. A 'good' mother is ever present with her children, so I felt guilty for working. This isn't good guilt. Working isn't a behaviour I'm not proud of, it's not something I want to amend, so it can't be guilt. Instead, it must be me measuring myself against someone else's standards. Psychologist Dr Rick Hanson told me, 'Guilt involves two things: some kind of standard plus a perception that we're falling short of that standard. That gap, that shortfall, produces feelings of guilt. So then the question becomes: What are fair standards for yourself? Very often, we feel guilty because we've internalized unreasonable, inappropriate, unfair standards from the culture, from our partner, from our parents, from our boss, or from the relatives – but they do not have to be your *own* standards. You can decide for yourself what it means to be a good-enough mother.'

I feel discomfort when I don't live up to the cultural pressure of what a 'good' mother should be, but it's not guilt. I always feel uncomfortable when I act in a way that's not expected of me, because doing life on our own terms *is* uncomfortable. It would have been much easier for me to keep my head down and carry on in my corporate job, but instead I started a podcast about modern mother-hood because that was how I wanted to show up in the world. It was uncomfortable to start with, but it wasn't guilt. And it isn't guilt when you leave an unhappy marriage to finally find the love you deserve (and show your children what that looks like) – it's the discomfort of not doing what's expected of you. And it's not guilt when you decide to put your children into a school where there's no uniform or curriculum and your whole family judges you for it – it's the discomfort of not doing what's expected of you. And it isn't guilt when you have a night away, so you can take a moment to breathe and ground yourself again – it's the discomfort of not doing what's expected of you. It's the discomfort of breaking cycles, but it's not guilt.

You can also feel discomfort when you do something you wouldn't have expected of yourself. In fact, feeling discomfort is usually a sign of growth. The moment we step outside our comfort zone, we will feel discomfort. But it's not guilt, it's growth. You decide to rest on the sofa before school pick-up, because you're exhausted and you want to be present for your children, but the moment you sit down you feel 'guilty'. That's not guilt – it's discomfort at breaking your pattern of rushing until you break. It's the discomfort you feel at living your new value of caring for yourself.

Remember, we are living in an era of 'intensive mothering' (see page 68) where the cultural memo we've been passed is that we need to be *everything* to our children. It's no wonder 94 per cent of us feel guilty, because being everything is an impossible task.[45]

> **Motherkind Moment**
> We've set ourselves an impossibly high bar and feel guilty every time we fall short.

We don't need to 'try harder', we need to lower the bar. You get to decide which bars to lower. Founder of Pregnant Then Screwed Joeli Brearley told me, 'Guilt is a man-made issue, in that we are constantly told to feel guilty as women. Men are not told to constantly feel guilty. Very often headlines in newspapers do that to women, they purposefully twist things as if it's our fault.' One of the greatest acts in motherhood is to define your own values and standards. Ask yourself, 'What is really important to me and my family?' Dr Rick Hanson told me, 'You have the right to define your job description, to claim it for yourself – you get to decide that.'

One of the greatest acts in motherhood is to define your own values and standards. Ask yourself, 'What is really important to me and my family?'

Figure out which standards you want to drop, then, step-by-step and day-by-day, start acting on this. Of course there will be discomfort. Of course you will question yourself. But don't call it guilt. Instead, celebrate these feelings because they represent growth. The more we act in line with our own values, the more discomfort we feel. The more we grow into ourselves and do what's not expected of us, the more we have to learn to live with feelings of discomfort. Discomfort is an expected passenger of a motherhood well lived.

A group of psychologists in the Netherlands wanted to understand why mothers felt more guilty than fathers when they went to work. They discovered that internalized ideas of what a 'good' mother does versus a 'good' father was driving the amount of guilt felt. This proves that it's our internalized beliefs and standards that create so much guilt. But we can change this.[46]

> **Motherkind Moment**
> I am allowed to define my own standards. The discomfort I feel is growth, not guilt.

> **Motherkind Toolkit: I should …**
> Remember the 'should sham' exercise on page 33? It's important here because whenever you hear 'I should', it is usually a sign that you are measuring yourself against someone else's standards. Notice whenever you hear 'I should' and ask yourself: 'Whose standard is this? How do I feel about my actions?'

Inner critic

If you've picked up this book, then I know that you want to enjoy motherhood, raise resilient, kind children, and be a wonderful mother. I've never cared about anything more than I care about my children. I've never felt so invested in anything as I do in raising my girls. I also have a very strong inner critic and the more I care about something, the louder that critic becomes. My critic has always told me I'm awful, but I'd never noticed it as brightly before. It's like motherhood took a highlighter pen to my lack of empathy for myself. So, it's no wonder that internal voice telling me 'I'm not doing it right' is really loud in parenting. We introduced the inner critic in Chapter Two; let's learn how it impacts on guilt and what we can do about it.

When I first started having therapy I was afraid the therapist would find out my deepest fear: that I was an awful, flawed human who didn't deserve anything good. I actually found out the opposite and continue to discover that I (like you) am a wonderful, loving, kind human who deserves all the good in the world. Children are such a gift, especially if you've had a challenging journey to motherhood. But the gap between your feeling of worthiness for your children and your love for them is where your inner critic can get really loud. If deep down you feel undeserving of your children, then it's likely your inner critic criticizes you for even the smallest perceived failure: 'Oh, pasta again, is it? Don't you know anything about nutrition?' You can't win against your inner critic. It will criticize you for serving pasta again, then when you serve something else it will tell you, 'What's the point? You know they won't eat it and you're just going to upset them.' This voice isn't a rational one. It isn't one to argue with, because you can never win.

Dr Nicole LePera told me that what we've thought of as our inner critic is actually our inherited critic. The harsh voices we hear in our heads aren't ours at all, but criticisms we absorbed in our early years (when our brains were like sponges so we heard everything as truth). These criticisms could have been from parents, caregivers, or even societal messages we absorbed. So, if we were guilted or even shamed in our childhoods ('What's wrong with you?' 'Why can't you do anything right?' 'Why do you never listen?') then that voice could become our inner critic. We don't even need the critical messages anymore; we do it to ourselves.

My client Ava was criticised for not tidying up enough as a child. 'You're so spoilt,' her parents would say. 'Look at all these toys – tidy them up now, or else up to your room with no dinner.' She had absorbed that she was lazy and struggled to care for her things as her truth. Now fast forward thirty years, she's a mother of two and lives with constant guilt for not having a tidy enough house, even though she tells me it's pretty spotless. Ava's brain is trying to protect her from hurt (remember our brain's primary function is safety) from perceived criticism, and the best way it knows how to do this is to be extremely critical to keep in her line. Freedom for Ava came when she realized where this constant guilt was coming from. Now she acknowledges her inner critic, thanks it for trying to keep her safe, reminds herself she's an adult now, and is learning to hear the voice but not listen to it.

> **Motherkind Moment**
> We can't control the thoughts that come into our minds; I have guilty, critical, and shaming thoughts most days. But we can control what we do with these thoughts.

The greatest skill I have learned is to not make my thoughts my reality. A thought only has power if we believe it. So, my first thought may say, 'You're lazy for sitting down when the house is a mess,' but I recognize that this is my inner critic and choose not to change in my actions (remember the first thought, second thought tool from page 55). I don't make a critical, negative thought right and my conscious mind wrong. I can choose to stay sitting with my cup of hot tea. And the more I've been able to do this, the easier it becomes.

Mindfulness is often misunderstood. It's not about thinking only positive thoughts or stopping unwanted thoughts entirely. It's about learning that you are not your thoughts. It's about being able to create space and choice.

The other day my daughter poured a packet of sweets onto the table. 'I only want the pink ones,' she said. That's the skill of mindfulness – it's being able to pick which thoughts you listen to and which ones are going to hold you back or make you feel bad. You can develop the skill of being able to pick the pink ones by focusing on what you want, how you want to behave, and what is good. This gives you choice over the thoughts you want to make your truth.

Motherkind Toolkit: Challenge your guilt thoughts
Practise noticing your thoughts without automatically believing them. Practise saying the mantra; 'I don't have to believe every thought I have.'

Permeating

Remember that time I really wanted to go to my breathwork class (where I get to scream into a pillow without anyone questioning my mental health: hard recommend) but the girls were begging me to stay at home? 'I want a Mummy bedtime,' my three-year-old was screaming over and over. My hypervigilance meant that I could see my husband's face changing as he became more frustrated and worried about getting the girls to bed. He didn't need to say a word and yet I took on his feelings. So low was my capacity for anyone to be annoyed at me that the first time this happened I decided not to go. And I was furious with myself, my husband, and my kids. But it wasn't their fault. I'd taken on their feelings as my own and allowed them to change *my* actions. I had a huge breakthrough when I realized that no one had the power to 'make' me feel guilty: I was doing that myself by allowing someone else's feelings to permeate my own. That night I was snappy with the girls, resentful of Guy, and it was all on me.

The following month I was sitting with Dr Becky, clinical psychologist and founder of parenting platform Good Inside. That experience was still bothering me, so I asked her: 'Why do I feel so guilty when I try to do something for myself?' Her answer was animated and quick: 'We've been taught to take in other people's distress and transform it into *our guilt,* and then once it's our guilt we have the responsibility to rework it instead of the other person.' Dr Becky says our ability to have our needs met, and to care for ourselves, depends on developing the skill of not taking on others' distress at our actions. And this was a skill I definitely needed to develop. I was waiting for everyone around me to be happy about meeting my own needs; 'Never going to happen,' quipped Dr Becky.

Dr Becky shared with me a brilliant analogy of a tennis court that I use most days. I imagine me on one side with a need or thing I want to do, and I imagine the other person on the other side with their feelings about it. There's a piece of glass between us, so I can see and hear them, but their feelings can't become my own. I am free. Just like my embarrassing forehand, it takes practice to not take on others' feelings. I still do, of course, but even when this happens, I'm aware of what I'm doing and that is half the battle won.

A few weeks later, and it's the same scenario. It's the night of my breathwork class, and the girls are begging me not to go. I take a deep breath, remind myself these are not my feelings, I have nothing to feel guilty about, and I am building resilience in them by going. Two things are true: I'm a good mother AND my children are sad that I'm leaving. I go to my class, take some deep breaths, scream into a pillow, cry in meditation, and come back feeling renewed. The next morning my eldest said to me, 'Mummy, did you have a lovely class? We had such a good time with Daddy.'

Motherkind Toolkit: Are your feelings your own?
Notice when you are taking on other people's feelings as your own. Ask yourself, 'Is this my feeling or someone else's?'

Shame

Brené Brown, author of *The Gifts of Imperfection*, teaches that guilt is 'I feel awful', whereas shame is 'I am awful'. Guilt is about the outside, i.e. what you did; shame is about the inside, i.e. who you are. Brené writes that shame is a paralysing emotion, a 'deeply painful experience of believing that we are flawed and somehow unworthy – I am not enough'.

Much of the 'guilt' we experience as mothers is actually shame. We feel like bad mothers for working, for not working, for not wanting to play another game, for forgetting to pack the right sports kit. It's not about our behaviour at all: it becomes about who we are.

As psychologist and author of *A Manual for Being Human* Dr Soph Mort told me, 'Shame is like having an open wound and then pouring salt into it.' We *feel* bad and then we double down in that feeling by deciding we *are* bad. Here's the difference between guilt and shame: good guilt is: 'I shouted at my kids too much today, because I'm tired, worried about work, and stressed. I'll apologize to them at bedtime and make sure I get an early night tonight.' Shame is: 'I shouted. I'm a terrible mother.' With good guilt there's room for compassion and change; with shame we write ourselves off.

> **Motherkind Moment**
> If you find yourself saying, 'I am …' that's a clue that you're in shame.

Feeling accepted and understood is what stops the shame. I witness this time and time again when I coach groups of mothers. Someone's most shameful thoughts – 'I'm not sure I'm cut out for motherhood', 'Some days I fantasize about my childfree life', or 'I feel like running away' – are met with nothing but understanding and kindness. Strength comes from knowing you are not alone, and there is nothing wrong with you. Therapist and author of *Wise Words for Women* Donna Lancaster told me, 'There's something about speaking our shame out into the world that is so healing for other women to hear, other mothers in particular to be able to say: "Yes, me too." That is how we heal our shame: we share it with others who will not shame us.'

> **Motherkind Toolkit: Share your shame**
> Is there someone safe you can share your shame with? If you can't think of anyone, go into nature: find a beautiful tree or a river and tell it. Imagine being fully accepted and loved.

Is it guilt or grief?

One of the biggest gifts of speaking to incredible, wise experts on the *Motherkind* podcast is that every week I learn something new, I see something differently, I change my mind and my perspective, and I reflect. But this is also one of the hardest parts as I'm constantly realizing where I've missed the mark in the past. I've grieved the hours and weeks lost to self-loathing when I didn't know any better. I've cried tears of regret for not knowing what I now understand about my baby's developing brain. I've felt the sting of shame when thinking about what a martyr I was during the early years of motherhood. I've wanted to go back and shake my younger self when she didn't know to set boundaries, advocate for herself, or give herself a break. I've mourned those early months when I didn't understand matrescence. I've had to become an expert in self-forgiveness.

But we can't judge our past selves with the knowledge we have now. We can't judge the person we were two years ago, two months ago, or even two days ago, because we're ever evolving and we're different now. I send that version of me love; she was trying her best with what she had, just like the present me is. I have Maya Angelou's words on my office wall, enveloping me with their kindness:

'Do the best you can until you know better. Then when you know better, do better.'

MAYA ANGELOU

Growth is a double-edged sword. It brings new awareness and knowledge as we inch ever closer to more joy, self-acceptance, and ease. But at the same time, we can feel guilt, or even grief, that we didn't get there sooner, that we didn't know then what we know now. Listeners to the podcast with older children often tell me, 'I wish *Motherkind* had been around when my children were little, how different it might have been.' And I always reply with: 'Trust that you were meant to learn, when you learned it, right on time, not a minute before or a minute after.' I have had to remind myself of this so often that I wear a bracelet with the word 'trust' on it. It sits on either side of bracelets with my girls' names on. I'm glancing down at it now as I remember I can trust myself, I can trust that I'll learn what I'm meant to right on time. And my shoulders drop a little. That five-letter word has released me from the bind of guilt, shame, and regret more times than I count.

Donna Lancaster told me about her experience: 'My grief work was around the fact that I don't remember significant events in my early children's lives. I don't remember baby teeth coming out for the first time, I don't remember birthdays, I don't even remember early Christmases because I was traumatized. I was in survival. So, I did what was necessary to keep my children clean and healthy and safe, but I was in a trauma trance. So that grief, to actually feel the sadness, is fundamental for me to process it.'

Maybe some of the things we feel most regret for will be the very things that form our children into who they are meant to be. My mum once told me she feels extremely guilty about some events in my late teens, but I see it differently. If I hadn't had those experiences, I would never have sought therapy, trained as a coach, and ultimately started Motherkind, which has changed my life. I am a better person because of her 'mistakes'. I have experienced personal growth on a level that wouldn't have been possible otherwise. What she feels guilty about, I feel grateful for.

I was holding my first born in my arms when I realized I wanted to write my mum a letter, thanking her for everything she'd done for me. I wanted her to be free of guilt and regret. I wanted her to know that even with her imperfections, even with her struggles, I was grateful. She told me that she fell to the ground when she read it, sobbing, releasing decades of guilt. She told me she felt free after that day. I didn't want my incredible mum to spend another minute feeling guilty – I wanted her to focus on what she did for me, not on what she didn't. And I want that for you too.

> **Motherkind Moment**
> We have to start believing that we're doing the best we can with what we've got.

Your new superpower: your values

Not knowing our values in motherhood is like driving to a destination without having any idea where our destination is. Values are our compass and map: they help us make choices, be able to differentiate 'good guilt' while turning down the volume on others' opinions and live a life that feels more fulfilling and aligned to who we really are. I think of values as a set of guiding principles. And if ever we need our own guidance, it's in motherhood.

Values are meant to change as life changes, so it's vital we update our values as our families grow and change. Having clarity on my values has meant I'm able to stand firm in my decisions and choices. It means being able to make more intentional choices, learn to listen to my own voice, and, crucially, feel less guilty. It's like leaves and trees – when I wasn't clear on my values in motherhood, I felt like a leaf being blown around on the winds of other people's expectations, judgements, and standards. Now, having absolute clarity on my values, I feel more like a tree: firm, strong, steady. Relationship expert and author Paul C. Brunson told me that 'a lot of us, what we do is we think about what we would like to value or what our friends and family would like us to value. And then we list those as our values. But instead, look at where you spend your excess time and your excess money as an adult, that's really where your values lie.'

Motherkind Toolkit: Define your values

This exercise, called Peak Experience, will help you to define your values in just fifteen minutes:

1. Choose an experience in your life when you've felt peak joy and happiness, when you felt totally in flow and at peace, and there was no struggle or self-doubt. It could be a brief moment or a longer experience. Try not to overthink what you choose; you can always repeat the exercise a few times. Clients have chosen their wedding morning, a moment at a music festival, the feeling of sun on their face at sunrise, or jumping on the bed with their children.
2. Write about the experience or talk it out to yourself. Try to connect to the emotion you felt at the time.
3. Now have a think about what values you were living in that moment – circle the ones from the table overleaf that fit.

Authenticity	Growth	Recognition
Achievement	Happiness	Reputation
Adventure	Honesty	Respect
Authority	Humour	Responsibility
Autonomy	Influence	Security
Balance	Justice	Self-respect
Beauty	Kindness	Spirituality
Compassion	Knowledge	Stability
Community	Learning	Success
Creativity	Love	Status
Curiosity	Loyalty	Trustworthiness
Determination	Meaningful Work	Wealth
Fairness	Optimism	Wisdom
Friendships	Peace	
Fun	Pleasure	

4. From those circled, think about your top five to ten values and jot them down. Do these feel right? Remember to choose your actual values, not the ones you think you 'should' have, and remember that your values can change over time as you grow. What you value now will be very different from what you valued in your younger years. Once you've got your list, put it somewhere visible (mine are on the fridge) – values are meant to lived, not shoved in a drawer and forgotten about. Paul C. Brunson told me, 'The test to determine if those are truly your values is that the more you live that value the more you light up.'

5. If you want to take this tool a step further, score your values against how you feel you are living each one, where zero is not at all and ten is feeling a connection most days.

6. Choose one value to focus on and ask yourself:
   - How could I live this value more in my life?
   - How would my life feel if I was living this value at a ten every day?
   - What changes would I make from where I am today?
   - What decisions might I need to make differently?
   - What is one small change I can make this week to live more in line with this value?
7. Repeat the exercise with your partner, co-parent, other caregivers, and children. Choose a moment you shared as a peak experience.

Let's transform your relationship with guilt

What if we didn't constantly judge our own mothering skills? What if we could learn to embrace good guilt but stop our shaming, judgemental inner critic before it stops us feeling the joy, presence, and esteem we deserve? When we're standing over ourselves, clipboard in hand, constantly writing an 'F' next to our best efforts, it makes us overwork, overgive, overcompensate, and push our needs even further down the pecking order. We become stuck in a shame spiral: we tell ourselves we're not good enough, so we try harder and push ourselves more until we're exhausted. And then we repeat the cycle. This stops us asking for help. It stops us questioning the system we mother in. It keeps us small and stops us advocating for ourselves.

The key to transforming our relationship with these challenging feelings is to take ownership of them. The worst thing we can do is ignore our feelings, thinking they don't matter. Because they do – your experience of motherhood matters.

Motherkind Moment
You will be a mother until the day you die, so it's worth learning how to navigate your most difficult emotions about motherhood.

It's true that 'What you resist, persists.' The more I tried to ignore my guilt and push it away, the worse it got. Because putting your metaphorical fingers in your ears and humming doesn't make the feeling go away; it only pushes it underground, further into your psyche. Whenever you feel guilty, use the flow chart opposite to instantly reframe it.

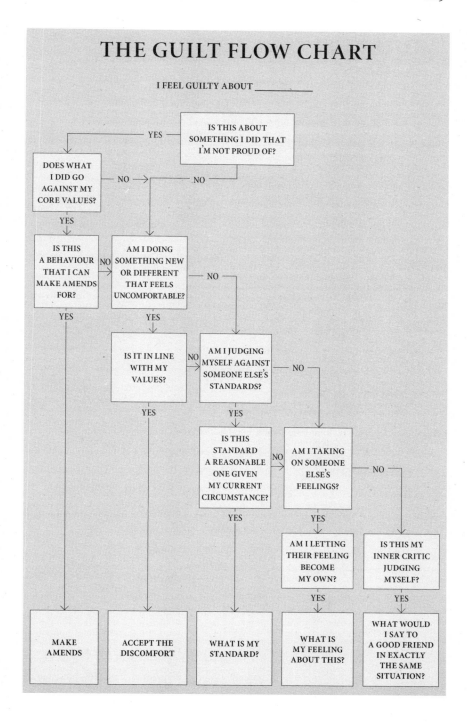

THE GUILT FLOW CHART

I FEEL GUILTY ABOUT _____

IS THIS ABOUT SOMETHING I DID THAT I'M NOT PROUD OF?

YES

DOES WHAT I DID GO AGAINST MY CORE VALUES?

NO

NO

YES

IS THIS A BEHAVIOUR THAT I CAN MAKE AMENDS FOR?

NO

AM I DOING SOMETHING NEW OR DIFFERENT THAT FEELS UNCOMFORTABLE?

NO

YES

YES

IS IT IN LINE WITH MY VALUES?

NO

AM I JUDGING MYSELF AGAINST SOMEONE ELSE'S STANDARDS?

NO

YES

YES

IS THIS STANDARD A REASONABLE ONE GIVEN MY CURRENT CIRCUMSTANCE?

NO

AM I TAKING ON SOMEONE ELSE'S FEELINGS?

NO

YES

YES

AM I LETTING THEIR FEELING BECOME MY OWN?

IS THIS MY INNER CRITIC JUDGING MYSELF?

YES

YES

MAKE AMENDS

ACCEPT THE DISCOMFORT

WHAT IS MY STANDARD?

WHAT IS MY FEELING ABOUT THIS?

WHAT WOULD I SAY TO A GOOD FRIEND IN EXACTLY THE SAME SITUATION?

If you only have five minutes today ...

- Guilt is an overused term in motherhood, and often disguises what is actually happening.
- Good guilt is when we act outside our values in a way we're not proud of and feel driven to reflect and make amends.
- Good guilt is welcome. It helps us form positive, intimate relationships.
- About 20 per cent of what we label guilt is good guilt. The other 80 per cent is a mixture of expectations, our inner critic, messages we have absorbed, and shame.
- When we fall short of our internal or external expectations of ourselves, we feel discomfort. But this discomfort is actually growth that we need to learn to accept.
- Our inner critic gets very loud in motherhood because it matters so much.
- We need to learn not to believe every thought we think. Using mindfulness tools can guide us.
- When we take on the feelings of others as our own, we feel discomfort. We can develop the skill of tolerating others' disappointment in our actions.
- Guilt is 'I feel awful', shame is 'I am awful'.
- When we experience shame, we keep ourselves stuck.
- We can learn to trust our path through motherhood, and have compassion for our regrets and what we wished we'd done differently.
- We all deserve our own compassion and understanding.
- Knowing our unique values is key to feeling positive about ourselves and our choices in motherhood.

Chapter Nine: Boundaries, not balance

'Boundaries are like fences; they keep out what you don't want and protect what you value.'

HENRY CLOUD, AUTHOR OF
Boundaries: When to Say Yes, How to Say No, to Take Control of Your Life

Balance in motherhood is a myth. There, I've said it. I've tried to find the perfect balance, where all the important things in my life are given a balanced amount of time, energy, and attention, and it never happens. I've never found that elusive time when I've felt no tension between work, home, and my needs. It just doesn't exist. *There is always tension.* So, let's burst the balance bubble and set ourselves free from feeling like we're failing all the time. Let's focus on what does work: *boundaries.* This means setting limits in every area of your life, including with yourself for what you need and what works for you.

It's okay if you have no idea what I'm talking about right now. When I first heard the word 'boundaries' from a therapist, I wondered why she was talking about neighbours and garden fences (I had only heard that word before to describe a party wall dispute).

> **Motherkind Moment**
> Boundaries are how you decide and then communicate what's okay
> and not okay for you. Boundaries are a way of recognizing you're
> not limitless.

You are not an endless well of giving and doing, and meeting everyone's needs around you but your own. You do not have to fit in with your mother-in-law's plans when they don't work for you. You do not have to socialize when you're exhausted just because your partner wants to. You do not have to talk about something that is too painful because someone asked you about it. You have limits. You have limits for how much you're able to give, for what makes you feel safe, and for how people come into your life, home, and emotions. Telling yourself and others about these limits is what creates boundaries.

There are two types of boundaries: the first is the external limits we set with other people, and how we communicate what is okay and not okay for us. The second is internal boundaries, which are the limits we set with ourselves and our own behaviour. In motherhood both these types of boundaries are absolutely vital; without them we'll exhaust ourselves physically and emotionally, and feel annoyed, taken advantage of, or even resentful of the people around us.

> **Motherkind Moment**
> Internal boundaries are the boundaries we hold with ourselves;
> external boundaries are those we hold with others.

I often think about paddling pools when I think about boundaries. Imagine you're starting to meet your own needs – you might be drinking enough water, going to bed earlier, and eating well;

you're filling up your paddling pool. Then imagine you don't have boundaries, so the moment someone asks something of you, you say yes. You might even offer to do things you don't really want to in an attempt to be liked. You might answer a call to someone you don't really want to speak to, then feel guilty for being cold and curt. This is like having no sides in your paddling pool – every time you fill it up, it drains away and leaves you empty.

That's how it feels to need more boundaries in your life – that no matter what you do, you can't catch up with yourself. You might end up doing things you don't really want to do, find yourself drawn into dramas you don't want to be involved in, maybe even in friendships you don't really want to be in anymore. You might find yourself biting your lip as you watch your parents do something with your children you've repeatedly asked them not to do. Or you might be building up serious resentment against your colleagues because you keep having to pick up extra work. Almost every client I've ever worked with has struggled with setting boundaries, and yet learning to say no, prioritizing our energy, and becoming intentional about our choices is the foundational skill we need in modern motherhood.

Why is setting boundaries so uncomfortable?

I tried to speak clearly and kindly to hide the slight wobble in my voice as I said the words, 'Thank you so much for inviting us all to lunch. I really appreciate the effort and thought but I'm not going to come with you all today.' I paused with bated breath, watching for every inflection on my father-in-law's face as I waited for a response. 'No problem,' he said. And that was that. I felt a rush of pride as I'd had the courage to share my inner truth – that I didn't want to go to lunch – outwardly. This might seem like a laughably small thing to do, but for a recovering people pleaser like me, it's massive.

For most of my adult life I've been invested in two things: keeping the peace and keeping others happy. I would rather risk hurting myself than others. So that afternoon, knackered from six months of sleep deprivation and yearning for some space to myself, I did something different. I risked hurting my father-in-law's feelings in order to value my own. It felt uncomfortable. In fact, the courage it took to do this felt hugely disproportionate to the situation. Pushing your needs towards the top of the pile and setting boundaries is hard.

Melissa Urban, author of *The Book of Boundaries: Set the Limits That Will Set You Free*, told me, 'We have been conditioned to not have needs when we become mothers. We are praised the most when we are selfless – when we have given up ourselves for the sake of our children. And when we do have a need, and express it, we're told we're selfish. We're told we're too controlling, and we have too many rules. So, we've learned not to have needs, and if we do have them, certainly don't speak up about them. There is a huge unlearning that has to happen before we can feel comfortable advocating for ourselves in the form of boundaries.'

Remember on page 138 we discussed 'good girl' conditioning? Well, this is another way it plays out. As women, we have absorbed from an early age that to be 'good' is to fit in, play nicely, go along with what others want, keep the peace, and not rock the boat. Now here we are as mothers, with impossible demands being placed on us – never-ending to-do lists, constant requests and pulls on our time – and we struggle to set the limits we need, firstly because we've never been shown how, and secondly because we're so afraid of not being seen as 'nice'. Terri Cole, author of *Boundary Boss*, told me, 'We were raised and praised for being self-abandoning.'

Motherhood doubles our to-dos and halves our time. This is why boundaries are a vital skill to learn in motherhood. Before mother-hood many of my clients already struggled with boundaries, but it didn't impact their lives too much. They could work until midnight for a demanding boss, go to dinners they didn't really want to be at, give more than they really wanted to, and often the only person really affected was *themselves*. Motherhood changes that because your time is no longer your own. And you have significantly less of it.

The great news is that having children to protect automatically flexes your limit-setting muscle. One client told me she had never spoken up to her mother before; as a well-conditioned 'good girl' she had never had boundaries. Until one day her mother was holding her newborn, who started crying. 'I'll take her,' my client said, gesturing to her mother to hand her back. 'No, no, I can settle her,' said her mother, slightly turning away. My client didn't know what came over her as her voice became loud and clear, she marched over to her mother, took back her unsettled baby and sternly said, 'She needs ME.'

When my eldest daughter was a newborn I attached a sign, written in thick black ink, on our front door: 'DO NOT KNOCK, baby sleeping.' I would never have done that before becoming a mother, as I was too scared to seem rude to the delivery person, to passers-by, to visitors, but now I would do anything to stop our dog barking and keep my baby sleeping. That need was greater than my people-pleasing tendencies. And so it begins. Motherhood was the beginning of me finally learning to set boundaries, to meet my own needs, and state what works for me in my relationships. And guess what? The world kept spinning, I didn't become a horrible person, there weren't awful fights, but I did get back more time and energy.

Examples of boundaries with a newborn

- We're not allowing visitors to kiss the baby, but she loves to be held.
- We're not sharing pictures on social media, so please don't either.
- We're having the first five days just us in our bubble, then we'd love you to come over and meet him.

- Thanks for the advice, but I'm enjoying finding my own way in motherhood.
- I found the birth really hard, and I'm not ready to discuss it yet.
- We're doing sleep this way, because it feels right for us at the moment. It might change, but right now I'd be so grateful if you could support us in our choices.
- What I really need is practical support, not advice. What would really help is if you could possibly hang up these Baby-gros for me.

Examples of boundaries with grandparents

- We're choosing not to do time-outs based on the latest studies on child development, so please can you follow our rules and do this instead.
- I need some warning before you pop in to see us. Please could you call before you come to see if it's a good time.
- I've been researching the best nutrition for toddlers, so we're going to limit sugar for a little bit longer. Please don't buy him sweets, but strawberries are his absolute favourite.
- It's so kind that you want to buy lots of presents, we really appreciate the thought, but we just don't have the space. I'd love us all to club together and buy one big present I think he will love.
- I know my sister and I do it differently, and I respect her parenting. Please don't compare us, it makes me feel really uncomfortable.

Examples of boundaries with friends

- I might take longer to reply at the moment, please don't take it personally.

- Can we not gossip about other mums? I just feel like we're all doing our best.
- I'm not drinking at the moment. I'm happy if you want to, but I'll bring this lovely new non-alcoholic drink.
- This is a difficult topic for me, can we talk about something else?

Examples of boundaries at work

- I can't answer emails after 6 p.m.
- I won't take that promotion for no extra pay to reflect the additional pressure and responsibility.
- I am entitled to X carer days, as per my contract.

How to work out your boundaries

It was the most intense time of my morning. Guy was getting ready to leave for work, shifting from foot to foot impatiently watching the baby as I was trying to shower, eat breakfast, and get myself ready for the day. Then the phone rang, and I felt a wave of anger come over me. 'I can't speak now,' I thought angrily to myself, but not wanting to seem rude, I answered the call. This happened over and over again. My mum kindly rang in the morning to see how the night with our eight-month-old went, but I would be rushed and curt when speaking to her as my dripping-wet hair soaked the bedroom floor. I was feeling frustrated with her, but then I realized she had no idea that this time didn't work for me. I was actually being really unfair by answering and then being rude. I needed a boundary.

I could have just not answered, of course, which would have been an indirect boundary. But I was committed to practising more honesty in my relationships and asking for what I needed. So that night I said to her, 'It's so kind when you call every morning, but it's the most stressful time of my day. Could you call after lunch? Then we can have a proper chat.' Mum's response was kind and understanding. Being more honest about your needs can actually improve your relationships because it removes the resentment, and no relationship feels good when there's dishonesty and frustration lurking in the background. You deserve to be honest about what works for you, and so do the people around you. Being honest with someone in this way is actually a sign of how invested you are in the relationship, to the point where you're willing to have a difficult conversation with them, even when it's uncomfortable.

> **Motherkind Moment**
> A sure sign you need a boundary is when you feel annoyed, frustrated, and resentful.

Once I've explained boundaries to my clients, the response is often a mix of fear, anticipation, and excitement. Fear at other people's reactions and how it might change things (remember that fear is always present with any change), anticipation of what might happen, and excitement at the time, energy, and peace of mind that they suspect is coming their way. I wonder if you're feeling the same. Even if this feels like a confusing and overwhelming idea, I want to reassure you that you already have these boundaries within you, just as my frustration signalled to me when my mum was calling at an inconvenient time.

That sting of resentment is signalling to you as you pick up another child from school, even when it really inconvenienced you. As is that tightening in your chest as you agree for your partner to go away this weekend, even though you desperately need the support at home. And that frustration you feel when you agree to something that stretches you beyond your limits. They are all signalling to you that you need a boundary. You *already* have your limits and preferences; you now have to make them visible to others.

> **Motherkind Toolkit: Boundaries**
>
> Have a think about your past week. When did you feel frustrated, resentful, annoyed, or taken advantage of? Jot these down (don't be surprised if there's lots), then ask yourself:
>
> - Is this something you can control? Could this be a boundary issue?
> - What might that boundary be? You might not know at this stage, and that's okay. Or you might have a few different ideas, also okay. Remember, you might be learning this skill for the first time.
> - Read on to learn how to set and communicate your boundaries.

Start small

It's so tempting to want to dive in with the biggest, hardest boundary first, especially if you're feeling fired-up to start protecting your needs. But please don't. My best advice, having coached mothers through thousands of different boundary scenarios, is to start small in low-risk, low-emotion situations with a low chance of a big fallout. Start by setting boundaries in your life with the little things: saying no to a request on the school WhatsApp group, telling your hairdresser you don't like the cut, or the barista that it wasn't the coffee you ordered. It's a good idea to start practising with people you don't have a close emotional relationship with.

One of my clients is an incredible businesswoman and mother, but she struggles with boundaries. It really impacts her life as she often feels resentful and taken advantage of. She has a pattern of keeping quiet when she wants to speak up due to her people-pleasing programming and low self-worth. I suggested she start small, and life worked fast on giving her an opportunity to practise (as it often does). The next day she told me that she'd had a terrible haircut. She'd told the hairdresser she loved it with a fake smile plastered on her face, but walked away feeling angry and resentful at both herself for keeping quiet and at the hairdresser.

This is a sign that you're ready to change, that what you used to be able to brush off starts to bother you. It bothered her so much and she so wanted to break this pattern that after a week she took a deep breath, overrode her thoughts telling her it didn't matter, and called the hairdresser. The hairdresser was mortified and instantly offered to cut her hair again for free. So, my client went back to the hairdresser's, with every part of her wanting to run away. She had her hair redone and, luckily, was pleased with the second cut. But this wasn't about the haircut at all. This was about my client's desire to speak her truth, to be more honest, and value herself.

It was a massive breakthrough. She realized she could speak up and, far from being angry, the hairdresser was grateful she did so. She had started to rewrite a belief she had from 'It's better to keep quiet' to 'It's safe to speak my truth.' And this tiny action soon started to unlock her ability to speak up for herself in far more important areas of her life. Her self-worth grew and she began to feel more in control of her time. All from a bad haircut.

My client Laura found that as she explored her boundaries, they began to expand. She started by setting better work boundaries and surprised herself when she was soon also setting more boundaries with her partner. The benefits that she experienced from setting boundaries have also expanded. Setting and holding the boundaries she needed has created time for the activities she enjoys. She told me, 'The more I do, the more I continue to do.'

Fences, not walls

Boundaries aren't there to punish or to keep others away. Boundaries are for you, they are *your* limits. I once heard the phrase: 'Boundaries are fences, not walls.' We can change our boundaries, compromise on them, and open the gate sometimes. They don't need to be rigid; we don't need to become cold or distant with people in our lives to start using boundaries. In fact, when I started using boundaries in motherhood it brought me closer to many people, because I was finally being honest with how I felt and what I needed. I allowed my 'it's all fine' mask to drop and that vulnerability brought a deeper connection. Boundaries are often misunderstood as a weapon, to try to get others to change or to control their actions. But they aren't that at all, as you can never really change another person. Boundaries are about changing *your* side of the equation, changing what *you* do, in order to meet and respect your own needs and limits. And it doesn't mean you stop caring about others' needs; it means you start caring about your needs as well. It isn't all or nothing, them or you: it's both. You are sharing information about your limits and needs, and that doesn't need to be done harshly or rudely. Just like when we're told the rules of a game or the instructions for how to board the plane, it's just information.

Glass heads

My therapist once said to me when I was complaining about a friend not calling me when I was struggling: 'You know, Zoe, you don't have a glass head. People can't see what you need unless you tell them.' This was a lightbulb moment for me. My annoyance and resentment were triggered so often because I wasn't telling others what I needed and was then being resentful when they didn't do it. It's our job to communicate to others our limits, needs, and preferences, otherwise how are they supposed to know?

The three Cs of boundary communication

Once you have decided on a handful of boundaries you'd like to set, the next step is to communicate them.

1. Considerate

Like most things in life, when communicating a boundary, timing is everything. You're probably not going to get the result you want if you scream a boundary during an argument, or when emotions are high. Remember that boundaries aren't weapons; they are you communicating your limits. Before communicating a boundary, think about what the best time might be for both you and the other person. Depending on what the boundary is, and how important it is, think about whether it needs setting up beforehand, e.g. 'Can we talk about X later?'

When communicating your need, try to avoid using 'you' or blame statements; instead stick to 'I'. For example, 'Please can you not call in the morning because when you do that it stresses me out,' versus, 'I find it much easier to be present when we chat in the afternoon as I find it so hard to speak when I'm juggling a million things.' I also suggest never using the word 'boundary' when you're setting a boundary. I've done it a few times and it's never gone well, because 'boundary' can feel like therapy language. It can be perceived as having a superiority to it, and it sounds hard and harsh.

If you're new to communicating your needs, it's a really good idea to practise first. You don't want the first time you hear yourself say the words to be when the other person is in front of you. It might sound extreme, but jot down what you want to say and practise saying it in front of the mirror or with a friend. In the moment, you might feel nervous, so if you've practised then you give yourself the absolute best chance of getting the words out.

2. Clear

Brené Brown says that 'clear is kind', and hearing that changed how I felt about communicating boundaries. I used to think that it was kinder to smooth over the truth with, 'No, no, not a problem', or to pretend something didn't bother me, when it did. But now I understand that not being honest creates resentment in relationships. Imagine you're having coffee with a new mum friend, and she only agreed to meet you because she wanted to be 'kind', but she really didn't want to be there. In fact, the whole time she's thinking, 'I'm too busy for this', and maybe even resenting you for asking her. That would feel horrible, wouldn't it? Wouldn't you prefer her to be honest, and tell you she didn't have the time for coffee? I know I would. My friends often joke now that if I do something or say yes, they know that I really want to be there. Clear is kind.

When I first started learning how to communicate my needs I would overexplain, especially if there was silence. I would just keep talking and the more I talked, the less clear I became. There is so much power in stating your needs in as few words as possible and allowing there to be silences. Don't overcomplicate or overexplain; it's much easier for the other person if you keep it short. Clear is kind.

3. Compromise

Before you set a boundary, think about what you'd like to happen as a result. Do you want the other person to simply agree? To discuss it with you? Is this a non-negotiable or are you willing to compromise? Is what you're expressing a preference or a hard limit? It's really useful to have this clear beforehand, and you could even say, 'Yes, I thought you might say that, and I get why that would work for you. Would this work instead?' Remember that boundaries aren't walls or weapons, they are you asserting your needs and limits, and often there is compromise and flexibility within that.

You can also buy yourself time if the other person rejects your request or suggests something else. Some of my favourite phrases are:

- Let me think about that.
- I'm not sure how I feel about that, can you give me some time?
- I don't have an answer right now, can I come back to you?

Holding your boundary and learning to sit with the discomfort

When I first started setting boundaries, saying no and speaking up for what I needed was squirm-out-of-my-skin please-ground-swallow-me-up hard. Why? Because there is a direct link between boundaries and self-worth. A podcast guest once said to me, 'Boundaries are an external representation of our self-worth.' Which is why if you have low self-worth, you'll struggle with boundaries.

When I first started it went like this: I would set a boundary, the other person might question or challenge it, and I would cave. Why? Because I didn't feel the internal worth and strength to hold the boundary. I had a very unhelpful internal voice which said, 'Who are you to ask for what you want?' So, I would feel immense discomfort at prioritizing myself and that would lead me to say, 'Okay then, I will come,' or, 'Yes, you're right, it's not really a big deal.'

> **Motherkind Moment**
> The hardest thing about boundaries isn't setting them, it's holding them.

Starting to set boundaries in your life is uncomfortable, but feeling uncomfortable is a great sign that you have left your comfort zone (and your old conditioning of people pleasing) and are trying something new. But knowing that doesn't make it any easier, does it? My conditioning for making life easier for everyone else runs very deep. I've had to learn over the years to sit with the discomfort that comes with expressing my needs. Some therapists call that discomfort the 'afterburn': the feelings of guilt, fear, and anxiety we can experience when we start expressing our needs. This may be the first time we're beginning to own our power and take care of ourselves. Learning not to act on those feelings is how I learned to hold my boundaries and value my own needs. The more I was able to do that, the easier it got.

Don't let these feelings convince you that you are doing something wrong, because you're not. The feelings are signalling to you that this is hard because it's a new behaviour. When you first start using boundaries, you might feel like a 'bad person' because you're not used to valuing yourself in this way. But let me reassure you that you matter, your needs matter, and when you start expressing them, you will feel so much more empowered. The short-term discomfort of the 'afterburn' is worth the payoff of less resentment, and the extra energy and self-worth that you get from asking for what you need. Working with hundreds of mothers on setting boundaries in their lives, I've noticed a common pattern; those who struggle most tend to take too much responsibility for others' feelings. And an important part of the process is learning that you are not responsible for others' reactions to your boundary.

You are responsible for your reactions and behaviours, and other people are responsible for theirs.

Motherkind Community: Clare's story

On page 129 we met Clare, whose huge turning point came when she learned she wasn't responsible for other people's feelings, and it wasn't her job to make other people happy. Part of her transition involved putting boundaries in place. She began to say no to things that didn't work for her.

> 'Yes, it would be lovely to go out for Sunday lunch with my parents. But after a week of work and broken sleep due to teething, what I really wanted to do on Sunday was stay home in my pyjamas and watch a movie. I explored pausing to think about what I wanted and then asking for that.'

What if the other person reacts?

The key to boundaries is knowing that there will *always* be a reaction to your boundary. Accepting and expecting this makes it much easier. If people are used to us behaving in a certain way, they'll attempt to convince us to stay that way to avoid changing the dynamic. Often the reaction is defensiveness, and I know that when I've had boundaries set with me, that's often my first reaction too. I feel ashamed that I've 'done something wrong' and if that feels too much for me to hold, then I go to defence or even anger. So, it can help to expect a defensive reaction from the other person and prepare for it. And remember that, even though the other person will have a response, it is not your responsibility.

Motherkind Moment
Your responsibility is to communicate your needs, and the other person's reaction is their responsibility.

Sadly, you can't change others. You can't make people more emotionally mature; you can't make them respect you, or change. Your job is to hold your boundary, uncomfortable as it might be, and to show yourself and those around you that your words hold weight.

What if your boundary isn't respected?

This is the question I get asked most whenever I speak about boundaries and it's by far the hardest part. Most people in your life love you, want the best for you and your relationship, and you'll be able to work together to meet both your needs. But, unfortunately, this isn't true of everyone. So, what do you do when you've communicated your limit, considerately and clearly, you've tried to compromise, and yet still the boundary is ignored.

This is where you need to bring in the fourth 'C': consequence. Explain what you will do if this behaviour keeps happening. My client Marie had asked her parents not to let her two-year-old son watch YouTube when they were alone with him. She strongly felt it was inappropriate for him and set a non-negotiable boundary that she didn't want him to watch it, and she suggested other shows on his tablet she was happy for him to watch. After picking him up one day she realized he'd watched YouTube again, despite their assurance that they would respect her wishes. She was understandably upset.

Together we worked through what the possible consequences might be, and she decided that her best course of action was not to allow them to look after him until they agreed to respect her wishes. She was really concerned that her limit was being ignored and felt it was a broader safety issue for her. She told me her voice shook as she told them that was what she wanted to happen, and of course, they were shocked at her decision. But for the first time in her life, she felt empowered.

It's really hard to set consequences like this. It's hard deciding what they need to be and it's even harder to set and hold them, but sometimes, unfortunately, it's very necessary. For me, setting boundaries is the hardest part of my path to being a more empowered mother. It's also been where I've grown the most. Little by little I've changed from being an angry doormat – letting everyone walk over me and feeling rageful about it – to being someone who is willing and able to honour my needs, trust myself, and stand firm in my new belief that I matter.

> **Motherkind Toolkit: Setting consequences**
>
> - If your boundaries are being ignored, what might be an appropriate consequence?
> - What options do you have? Which one feels most aligned for you?
> - How will you communicate the consequence?

Boundaries with family

There's a famous phrase I love: 'Of course your family knows how to push your buttons, they are the ones that installed them.' The people who are closest to us also challenge us the most. Without a doubt, the majority of the boundary challenges my clients tell me about is with their family, usually siblings, parents, and in-laws. One client told me that just seeing her mother's name flash up on her phone made her chest tighten in anticipation of the criticism. We cannot control who we are related to, but we can control our reactions and put in place, using all the tools from this chapter, boundaries that feel right for us. It takes a lot of courage to start changing long-term patterns and dynamics in your family; it might take more energy than you have right now and that's okay too. You can start small and as your boundary muscle gets stronger, you can start to tackle the resentment and annoyances you have with your family.

When it comes to in-laws or wider family relationships, boundaries expert Melissa Urban taught me this brilliant principle on the podcast: 'You and your spouse have to agree on the boundary before you try to set it with either of your parents. Because if you don't, you stand no chance of holding the boundary together as a couple – and you could look like the "bad guy" for trying to enforce one at all.'

Melissa suggests the Numbers Game to quickly work out how important the issue is to both of you. Let's use the example of your five-year-old being given too much sugar by your parents: you might care nine out of ten about it because you're the one handling the meltdowns when they get back home. Your partner might be a three out of ten because they work through bedtime and don't have to navigate the tantrums. I love this quick little tool because it gives you a sense of where you both are on the issue. Now, Melissa advises, agree to the boundary based on the person with the highest score, because this issue is clearly more important to or impactful for them. Of course, this isn't easy – it takes practice and compromise – but it's an important principle and you have to be on the same page before communicating boundaries with family.

Learning to say no

The oldest, shortest words – 'yes' and 'no' – are those which require the most thought.

PYTHAGORAS

Learning to say no is such a power move in motherhood – your energy is so precious, you can't waste it on things you don't really want to do. I know it sounds obvious, but you can't do everything. Learn to say no to a playdate if you've already done too much that week. Say no to baking for the school fair if it's going to push you over the edge. Say no to meeting a friend if you know it's going to be too much that day. Say no to the extra work project if you know the impact it's going to have on your mental health.

What you don't do determines what you can do.

The challenge is, most of us have never learned to say no; we're too worried about what people will think. Will we be liked? Judged? Left out? We're so worried about what people will think that we risk our own feelings to avoid hurting someone else's. We might have FOMO (fear of missing out). We might think that if we say no, we'll never have another chance. We might hate conflict, or any risk of it, so we avoid saying no. We might have said no when we were younger and been criticized for it, so we learned to push down our real feelings and say yes anyway, even though we know the very real cost of doing that.

Costs can be financial – agreeing to host a gathering when you don't really want to, the cost of travelling to an event you don't want to be at, the cost of a wedding present for a wedding you don't want to go to, the cost of coffees on meet-ups you don't want to be at. Costs are also emotional: feeling exhausted, resentful, and frustrated with others and yourself. Perhaps you believe that saying no will make you a bad person? Let me bust that myth for you right now. There's a big difference between being nice and being kind. Nice is pushing down how you feel to seem a certain way. Nice is smiling on the outside, while seething on the inside. Nice is dishonest. Kind is when we give the other person the respect to be honest, and we trust that they have the maturity to handle how we really feel.

Saying no used to be so hard for me that I would do the opposite of a power move and push back the decision for another day: 'I'd love to but maybe next week,' and then it would niggle at me until next week came and I still didn't want to do it. Then sometimes I'd do that awful thing of cancelling at the last minute. What an energy drain for everyone involved. Here's my top tip: if you don't want to do it now, then you won't want to do it at a later date. Future you is no different to now you. Future you probably isn't going to have more energy, or suddenly start enjoying collecting money for the teacher's gift, or actually start liking that person. Learning not to kick the 'no' into the future is a gift to both you and the other person.

Motherkind Moment
Your time is the most precious resource you have, and you are allowed to say no.

Creating anything – a beautiful relationship with your child, a business, a new relationship, a stronger bond with your partner – requires focus, time, and energy, and you can only get this by saying no to other things that aren't as important to you. While I've been writing this book, I've said no so many times: to my children asking for me to do bath time, to friends asking me out for a coffee, to colleagues asking me to commit to events. Most of those things I've wanted to do, but I can't do it all. The idea that we can be it all and 'have it all' is a lie. You have to be clear on what your priorities are and make sure that your yeses and nos align with them.

How to say no

- Let me think about that (buy yourself some time: especially useful as you start developing this skill, then you can go back with one of the below).
- Thank you so much for inviting me, but I can't right now.
- That sounds amazing, congratulations and best of luck with it. I can't make it, but please do let me know how it goes.

- That sounds so fun, thanks for inviting me but I'm completely focused on work for the next three months.
- I have a rule of only one thing a day, so we can't come.
- I'm at my absolute capacity, so can't help I'm afraid.
- That timing doesn't work for us but thank you.

Boundaries with yourself

We've discussed external boundaries, those we set with others, but equally important are internal boundaries, those we set with ourselves.

> **Motherkind Moment**
> Internal boundaries are the promises you keep to yourself, to help you feel the way you want to.

How often do we sabotage our own best interests? We're exhausted but scroll on our phones way after our bedtimes. We're starving but grab a bag of crisps because we're too busy to eat properly. We're dehydrated but grab another coffee instead of a glass of water. I used to do this all the time until I learned about keeping promises to myself and that my word to myself matters. I learned that I matter, and I can show myself that through my actions. I also learned that I must look after myself if I'm going to be able to parent my children how I want to.

> **Motherkind Moment**
> Self-worth is not a feeling, it's an action.

We need to step in and become our own loving mother. We all know that parenting is about love *and* limits. In Chapter Two we learned about giving ourselves the love and compassion we need. Now we need to give ourselves the other side of the equation: limits. Psychologists call this 're-parenting', which means becoming our own parent.

> **Motherkind Moment**
> I am worthy of keeping promises to myself. I show myself I matter through my actions.

Just as with external boundaries, it's useful to start small. When discussing internal boundaries my client Jas shared how her toddler would shout for her every time she went to the bathroom. She would pee as quickly as humanly possible, give her hands a cursory splash, half pull up her trousers, and rush back out to her. She said she wanted to be able to go for a proper toilet break, wash her hands properly, straighten herself up and take a breath on her own before going back to her daughter. This is a tiny example, but such an important one because as mothers we tend to ignore our own (very) basic needs.

I asked Jas what came up for her when her daughter was shouting for attention. Jas broke down. When she was growing up her mother would spend long periods in the bathroom, and she had painful memories of waiting outside the door for her, crying. Jas desperately didn't want her daughter to experience the same feelings. We discussed how going for a two-minute bathroom break is very different to the forty-minute breaks she experienced with her own mother. It wasn't the same at all, but Jas's younger self was remembering the pain and reacting to it.

Sometimes when we have a painful memory we can experience

a pendulum effect and swing to the other extreme, as Jas was doing with her ten-second toilet breaks.

She committed to an internal boundary that she would allow herself a proper toilet break, taking at least a couple of minutes, and she had a great idea to get a special toy that her daughter could only have when she went to the toilet. This breakthrough, which all came from a tiny boundary, enabled Jas to look at all the other areas in her life where she was reacting from her past child rather than her present self.

Examples of boundaries with yourself

- I won't scroll through social media after 9 p.m.
- I'll aim to be in bed by 10 p.m. three times a week.
- I won't gossip about or judge other mums.
- I'll exercise three times a week.
- I won't check my phone first thing in the morning.
- I'll limit myself to three coffees a day.

Motherkind Toolkit: Internal boundaries

- What small promises do I want to make to myself?
- How will I encourage and support myself to keep my promises?
- How will I forgive myself and carry on if I break a promise?

If you only have five minutes today ...

- You are not limitless in how much you can give – recognizing those limits is called boundaries.
- Boundaries communicate what you need, and what is okay and not okay for you.

- There are two types of boundaries: boundaries with other people and boundaries with yourself.
- Boundaries help you take more control of your time, energy, and emotions, which is vital in motherhood.
- Boundaries can be challenging because we have been conditioned since childhood to be 'nice' and to 'fit-in' with others.
- In order to start meeting our own needs, we need to break this conditioning and believe that what we want matters.
- A sign of where a boundary is needed is if you feel taken advantage of, annoyed, or resentful.
- The key is to start small and practise on low-emotion, low-risk situations.
- The three Cs to communicating your boundaries are: Considerate, Clear, and Compromise.
- The hardest part of setting boundaries is holding them when others react. We may experience guilt or believe we have done something wrong. But we haven't.
- If your boundary isn't respected, you will need a consequence.
- Learning to say no is challenging if we have people-pleasing tendencies, but it's vital for protecting our time and energy.
- Learning to say no kindly and firmly is a skill we can develop.
- Boundaries with family are especially challenging because patterns can be so ingrained.
- Internal boundaries are the promises we keep to ourselves, to act in our own best interests, and are a form of mothering ourselves.
- Keeping a promise to ourselves is how we build our self-worth.
- Boundaries are challenging, but the payoff is feeling more empowered, and having less resentment and more authentic relationships.

Chapter Ten: Confident and capable

'No one can make you feel inferior without your consent.'

ELEANOR ROOSEVELT

My hands are shaking as I press record. I have no idea what I'm doing and as I speak, I can hear the shaky uncertainty in my voice. My chest flushes red and my stomach cramps with nerves. It's my first podcast recording, and it's awful. Come to think of it, many of my early podcast recordings were awful. I was a nervous host, spoke over the guest. I couldn't get the tech right. I asked obvious or confusing questions, and sometimes I spoke too much, other times too little.

You would have looked at me then, all trembles and insecurity, and perhaps not recognized the confident podcaster I have been able, through practice, to become. I still make more mistakes than I can count and have so much to learn, but I do have confidence. Of course, I still feel nervous before I press record, but I believe in my ability to keep trying, learning, and imperfectly showing up, and that's what I define as real confidence.

Almost every mother I know wants more self-confidence. So many mothers have come to me after experiencing a crisis of confidence in motherhood. Eighty-seven per cent of the Motherkind online community told me they didn't feel confident in themselves. So, if your confidence is wobbly, you're not alone. As we're going to explore, it makes sense that our confidence is lowered in motherhood when we understand how confidence is built.

Motherkind Moment
Confidence is our ability to keep imperfectly trying.

I believe we're all born confident, but our confidence becomes wrapped up in layers and layers of conditioning that makes us believe we're not good enough. Yet confidence is the skill that unlocks so much of what we've been discussing so far: asking for our needs to be met, setting and holding boundaries, trusting ourselves, believing in ourselves, asking for help, accepting help. We need confidence to ask for a pay rise, to ask for flexible working, to speak to the school about an issue, to have a hard conversation, to ask someone out for a coffee. We need confidence for almost everything in life, so why is it so misunderstood and elusive? Imagine if you could replace self-doubt with self-belief, if you could speak up when you need to, make decisions without overthinking, believe in your ability to mother your children, advocate for your children, feel secure and powerful.

I thought that confidence was something you either had or didn't have. Lucky for those that were born with it, unfortunate for those of us who, like me, have always doubted and questioned themselves. The Oxford English Dictionary defines confidence as 'a feeling of self-assurance arising from one's appreciation of one's own abilities or qualities'. One of the biggest myths is that confidence is a personality trait. In fact, it's a skill that can be learned and in motherhood we might have to learn this skill for the first time. Without a doubt, confidence is complex. It's built on layers of past experiences, traumas, race, and socio-economic status. And in motherhood our confidence is intertwined with our own experiences, neurodiversities, disabilities, and other challenges, but it's a skill we can all develop, and I'm going to show you how.

> **Motherkind Moment**
> Confidence is not a personality trait; it's a skill that can be learned.

> **Motherkind Musing**
> - What would having more confidence mean to you?
> - How would life be different if you had unshakable confidence?
> - What would you do differently?

The LEGO tower

Mothering is a learned skill, just like any other skill. Chelsea Conaboy, author of *Mother Brain*, told me, 'We are led to believe as mothers there is an unused part of our brain that suddenly gets turned on when we become mothers and that's called "instinct", which will mean that we know what to do, that mothering is easy and natural and innate. That is a *myth*. It doesn't come automatically; instinct comes through trial and error and time and it develops in response to our own particular children in response to their particular needs and to the social context around us.' I invite you to shake off any pressure you're putting on yourself that you 'should' know what to do. This is vital for developing confidence.

My confidence was at its lowest when I first became a mother. I had never even held a baby, let alone cared for one twenty-four/seven. As the days and weeks went on, I became more confident, getting to know my daughter and slowly building some muscle memory for the day-to-day out tasks. Then when she was six months old and it was time to start weaning, my confidence went back to zero. I had never fed a baby before. I was shaking as I handed her that first bite of solid food. After a few weeks my confidence grew, then it all changed again when she started walking. Again, my confidence was back to zero. This is the pattern of confidence; we build it up, then it lowers with every new age and stage.

Confidence is like a LEGO tower. It gets higher and higher as we add more bricks of experience, and as we grow our abilities as mothers. Think about the first time you tried to fold up your buggy. I bet it was awkward, it probably took you a while, there might have been swearing or, if you're anything like me, a quick YouTube tutorial on how to do it. Fast forward a few hundred times of folding it up and I'll bet you can do it almost without thinking, probably one-handed while also opening the front door and holding a child.

Motherkind Moment
Confidence builds through action.

One of the biggest myths about confidence is that you have to feel confident before taking action, as if confidence is a feeling that will magically come to you one day. If I waited until I felt confident to fold the buggy, I would never have tried. Confidence isn't a feeling to wait for, then take action; we take the action and then confidence builds. So, it's really the skill of *courage* we must develop first. We don't build the muscle of confidence when our experiences are familiar and comfortable; we build confidence when we experience the unfamiliar and uncomfortable.

Confidence is courage that has taken its first steps.

Five confidence myths busted

1. Confidence is the absence of doubt

We may look at a confident mother and instantly compare ourselves, assuming she has no doubts or insecurities. But think
about the moments when you have been most confident; doubt
and fear will still have been there, it's just that you decided to
act anyway. Confidence is not the absence of doubt, confidence
is trying anyway. I can't think of any time in my life when doubt
hasn't been present. Sometimes the volume is turned up high on
doubt and I have to work hard to find courage. Sometimes the
volume is lower, usually because of experience, and I can act
confidently with more ease. I cannot stress this enough: you can
be confident and doubt yourself. You can be confident and feel
scared. Confidence isn't the absence of fear and doubt, it's you
making a choice to act anyway.

2. Confidence is the same as extroversion

My idea of confidence used to be wrapped up in bravado, and very
externally focused. Now I know that version of confidence was
actually arrogance, masking insecurity and playing the role of what
I thought it meant to be 'confident'. For a long time, confidence has
been packaged up as the loudest in the room, showing no vulnerability or humility, often dressed in a power suit or standing on
a stage. At last, that version of confidence is changing, thanks in
part to the incredible work of author Susan Cain. In her bestselling
book, *Quiet: The Power of Introverts in a World That Can't Stop
Talking*, Susan explores how society has equated extroversion with
confidence for too long.

Lauren Currie OBE, founder and CEO of UPFRONT, told me,
'We don't need to aspire to what we think confidence looks like

in a patriarchal society.' People are often surprised when I say that I'm an introvert because I present as very confident, which I am in the true definition of the word. But unlike extroverts, being around people, presenting, or even going to parties drains me, and I need some time to recover afterwards. That is the key difference between introverts and extroverts – extroverts gain energy from being around people, whereas introverts might love to be around people just as much, but it leaves them with less energy.

3. Confidence is universal

We can feel extremely confident in some areas of our lives, and completely lack confidence in other areas. That's why the idea of a 'confident' woman is flawed – the reality is our levels of confidence will fluctuate depending on the level of experience we have in that area. The challenge with motherhood and confidence is that just as we gain experience with one stage or age, everything changes. Or just as we begin to feel confident with our working patterns, a child leaves or starts school and we have to re-adjust. Confidence can feel so low in motherhood because we are always stepping into unknown territory, which brings with it fear and vulnerability.

4. Confidence comes easily to women

How many times have you been told, 'Don't brag,' or heard, 'Who does she think she is?' Perhaps even from your family. I was very self-assured up until the age of nine – always singing and dancing, desperate to be an actress when I grew up. Then at school that all changed when the playground patter knocked me down a peg or two. These formative experiences with our sense of self have a long-lasting impact. It's taken me twenty years to build that confidence back to where it is today. Kasia Urbaniak, author of *Unbound: A Woman's Guide to Power*, explained to me that it's only in the last hundred years that it's been safe for women to speak up, and in many parts of the world it still isn't safe. So, as a survival mechanism women have learned to stay small, and this lives on in our collective memories and subconscious. Kasia also explained how our mothers may have tried to keep us small, polite, and not 'too big for our boots', because it was only a few generations ago that any behaviour other than this just wasn't acceptable for women.

We have to see our confidence as mothers in context, so we can have compassion and understanding for ourselves when we wobble.

5. A lack of confidence is our fault

Three powerhouse podcast guests, Reshma Saujani, Joeli Brearley, and Lauren Currie OBE, all told me the same thing: confidence is inextricably linked to our environment. Lauren is on a mission to 'change confidence, not women', because for too long women have been blamed for our lack of confidence, where in fact it's our environments that have hindered it. It's hard to feel confident when returning to work when we can hear the whispers of 'part-timer' from colleagues. It's hard to feel confident when you're told you're 'just a mother', or asked how your 'break' was when you return from maternity leave. It's hard to feel confident when the world doesn't value the invisible, life-forming, emotional work of motherhood. It's hard to feel confident when 54,000 women are pushed out of the workforce every year based on maternity discrimination. It's hard to feel confident when the motherhood penalty, as Joeli Brearley explained to me, means that on average a man will earn 21 per cent more when he becomes a father, while a woman will earn 30 per cent less when she becomes a mother.[47]

It's hard to feel confident when you're half as likely to be promoted when you work part time compared to full time. It's no wonder only one in five mothers feels confident when returning to work. It's hard to feel confident as a new mother when unsolicited advice is offered to you at every turn. So don't blame your lack of confidence on yourself – it makes complete sense in the confidence equation that the maths doesn't add up to you feeling confident and self-assured. So, let's ditch any self-criticism for your lack of confidence and begin working on what we can change right now: building your internal confidence, despite what's going on around you.

Motherkind Musing

- What do you need to unlearn about confidence?
- How has your confidence changed in motherhood?
- What abilities and qualities have you developed since becoming a mother?
- What can you do now that you couldn't do before becoming a mother?

Five ways to build unshakeable confidence

1. Expect and embrace fear

Fear is an unavoidable part of the human experience. Every single human on the planet experiences fear, and thank goodness for this, because fear keeps us safe; it stops us stepping out into the road or running towards danger. But this type of fear isn't the one we're going to talk about. The fear we need to understand if we want to feel more confident is the fear that holds us back, keeps us small, stops us asking for what we need or going for more. Have you seen the T-shirts saying 'fearless' in italics, or maybe the journals saying 'Fear has no place in your dreams'? Well, I need you to erase those messages from your mind because it's not true. Fear will be there, driving along with you in the passenger seat of your life, until the day you die. And the more you experience in life, the more fear will be present, because fear expands as you do. Remember, confidence isn't the absence of fear, it's acting even though fear is present.

The biggest trigger for fear is uncertainty. Just as for guilt (see Chapter Eight), it's important to make fear visible, because this brings more certainty into an action. When Guy and I were thinking about having a second child, we had endless conversations about it, going round in circles. Coincidentally, at the same time I was asked to feature on a radio programme about how to make the decision to have a second child or not. As I was prepping for the interview, reviewing my coaching tools, I realized that the tool we needed was Fear Setting. I learned this tool from podcaster and author Tim Ferriss, and it involves diving into the worst-case scenario, which is often the opposite of what we've been taught to do.

Motherkind Toolkit: Fear Setting

1. Choose a decision or situation you are not acting on (e.g. a new job, moving school or nursery, relocating, setting a boundary, ending or starting a relationship).

2. List everything you are afraid of, and the worst-case scenarios.

3. Note what you could do to prevent each scenario.

4. List ways you could fix the situation if the worst does happen.

5. Assess the impact of each of the worst-case scenarios, with zero being low impact and ten being life-altering.

6. Write down the best-case scenarios from the decision, remembering to capture the benefits of even a partial success.

7. Assess the impact of each of the best-case scenarios, with zero being low impact and ten being life-altering.

8. List the consequences of inaction over six months, one year, and three years.

We worked through the Fear Setting tool one evening and it was helpful to understand where we shared our fears and where they differed. We realized how negative our fears were, and actually fairly insignificant in comparison to the joy of bringing another person into our family. We started trying for another baby and sadly had two miscarriages along the way, but when our incredible youngest daughter was born it was and still is the best decision we ever made.

2. Start small, but start

The key to building your confidence is to start small. You can't think your way into being more confident, you have to act your way into it by leaning in to courage. Courage is walking into the toddler group when you feel anxious, uncertain, and worried if anyone will chat to you. It's applying for your first job after five years out of the workplace. It's calling the doctor when you're worried about your mental health. It's going for your first run in a decade. It's accepting the promotion even though you don't feel good enough.

Mel Robbins, author of *The 5 Second Rule*, told me we have five seconds to take action before our conscious, fear-based mind kicks in with all the reasons we shouldn't act. Many of my clients have used this tool to send an email to their boss with a request, to call a friend they've lost touch with, to get their trainers on and go for a run, or to finally have the mental load conversation. I taught my eldest daughter this trick and she used it the first time she jumped into the pool, when she doesn't want to start her homework, and when trying a new food.

3. Build confidence where you have none

We don't build confidence when something is easy; we discover what we're capable of when we do something new or hard. Every single client I've worked with has said some version of 'this is really hard, I feel out my depth'. And my answer is always the same: that feeling is a sign of growth. Change is uncomfortable because you are leaving your comfort zone and stretching yourself, and this builds confidence.

The learning zone

This learning zone model brilliantly visualizes that growth, and therefore confidence, comes from moving past what is comfortable and into the 'stretch' zone. Most of motherhood is spent in the stretch zone, so we need to get comfortable with the discomfort of it.

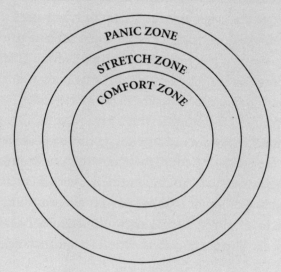

A diagram of 'The Learning Model' developed by John L. Luckner and Reldan S. Nadler (1991).

Setting a boundary? *Uncomfortable.*
Advocating for your needs at home? *Uncomfortable.*
Feeling your feelings instead of pushing them away? *Uncomfortable.*

That's why through this whole book I've suggested you start small, because change is effort and effort uses energy. We don't want to tip into the panic zone, which may happen if we decide that the first boundary we're going to set is with the CEO of our company, or plan a month-long trip with a baby when we've never even travelled alone before. You will know you're in the panic zone because it won't feel uncomfortable, it will feel unbearable.

4. Connecting with our younger selves

As Motherkind was growing, and I was becoming more visible, a part of me was excited and felt in my stretch zone. Then one day, someone sent me an offensive message and I panicked. I felt unsafe and afraid. I took a moment to ask myself, 'What part of me is afraid?' And I realized it was my younger self, or what psychologists call my inner child: the part of us still affected by experiences from our formative years (see page 283 for more on this). I realized that my inner child still felt so afraid of the school bullies, she wanted me to stay small to feel safe. (See page 166 for more about how our brain doesn't like change because it seeks familiarity, and Chapter Two to discover how our limiting beliefs about ourselves drive our behaviour.)

My client experienced this when she wanted to feel more confident speaking up at home and work. She realized that when she was growing up, she was punished and sometimes ridiculed for speaking up, and that this experience was stopping her from speaking up now. This is a crucial and often missed piece of the confidence puzzle. We have to welcome and mother that younger and perhaps scared part of us and offer support and compassion, just as we would with our children (I'll show you how on page 286).

Motherkind Musing

- When do you feel in your comfort zone? And stretch zone?
- How do you know if you're going into your panic zone?
- Is there a younger part of you that's holding you back?
- What does she need?

5. *Allow yourself to mess up and try again*

To develop confidence, you have to change your relationship with failure. We're going to fail at getting our children to eat all the vegetables and getting our babies into routines. We're going to fail at work, at that new fitness plan, and in our friendships. And we're going to fail our children. I know the last one stings, but we have to accept that failure and things not going how we'd like is part of showing up to life. We won't develop courage if we can't trust that if we fail, we'll be okay. On page 38 we discussed self-compassion and why it actually increases motivation. This is because if you know that you can try something, fail, and not be hard on yourself, you're more likely to keep trying.

At my kids' school they teach growth mindset right from the early years. There are posters everywhere saying, 'If I'm learning, I can't fail.' One of my favourite books on confidence is *Mindset* by Carol Dweck. Carol discusses that in a fixed mindset, the skills and ability to achieve are 'set', e.g. I'm not a confident person, I can't start my own business, I'm not a good mother, I'm not patient. A fixed mindset is the belief that we're either good at something or we're not, and no amount of effort will make any difference. So, if you have a fixed mindset, you don't even try, and this keeps us stuck. You might eye roll at a suggestion from a coach like me. You might decide 'I can't do that' without even trying or write yourself off as a stressed-out person who can't change.

I suspect, because you've picked up this book and got this far, that you have a growth mindset. With a growth mindset there is the recognition that skills grow with practice, and that almost everything in life is down to the effort you make. In this mindset, you know that practice is what builds skills, and that all skills can be worked on. The other day I was watching a television programme with my eldest daughter and one character said, 'I don't know how to bake a cake … yet.' This is a growth mindset. It's adding a 'yet' onto the limits you've put on yourself. Figuring out our path in motherhood is like trying to do algebra backwards blindfolded: it's hard. But a growth mindset reminds us, we *will* figure it out. There's nothing wrong with us, we're learning and trying and failing and learning again.

Motherkind Moment
My confidence isn't fixed: I can learn any new skills I need.

When I was in my early twenties, I heard the phrase: 'You can't fail, you win or you learn.' It changed my life. I decided that I would see everything in my life as a chance to learn about myself, about others, about the world. Sometimes the lessons are easy: I snap more when I let myself become depleted. And sometimes they are much harder to accept: a friendship ended because I wasn't honest enough about how I felt. But with a 'learning' mindset you remove a layer of self-criticism. 'I'm so awful, I messed that up' becomes 'I messed that up, but I learned something for next time.' I started seeing my actions as an experiment. I wondered what would happen if I spoke up, set a boundary, protected my energy, kept quiet, or tried a new parenting technique. And I took note of the outcome. It's a different lens to approach life, but it took the critical pressure off and made me far more likely to try new things.

I was once coaching a renowned university science lecturer who was really struggling with the stress and exhaustion of managing two young children with an intense job. We tried a few coaching techniques and tools, but it wasn't landing for her. So I asked her, 'What would you do if your stress was a scientific problem that you had to solve?' Her face changed. 'Easy,' she said. 'I'd come up with a hypothesis, I'd test it, then run test after test until I arrived at a conclusion.' When we 'fail', we're not failing at all; we're learning, as every experience gives us information.

Motherkind Moment
Every day is a chance to learn more about myself and my children. I am learning every day in every way.

Motherkind Musing
- What is your relationship with failure?
- Do you accept it as part of life or beat yourself up?
- How would life be different if you viewed your actions as experiments that you can learn from?
- What do you want to model to your children about handling failure?

A note on apologizing

I'm sorry she's crying.
I'm sorry I'm a mess.
I'm sorry the house is a mess.
I'm sorry we're late.
I'm sorry we can't make it.
I'm sorry I have to leave early.
I'm sorry the buggy takes up so much room.
I'm sorry I have to leave, the nursery just called.
I'm sorry I'm crying.
I'm sorry for asking.
I'm sorry for *existing*.

If one thing undermines our confidence as mothers, it's apologizing. Someone bumped into me yesterday; it was their fault, but I found myself saying, 'I'm sorry.' Women have been raised to apologize – it's in our DNA, like hating our bodies and pleasing everyone around us. Every time I apologize unnecessarily, I imagine myself taking a block off my confidence LEGO tower (see page 244), as apologizing chips away at our sense of worth. Try this little trick: instead of apologizing, say thank you. Thank you for your patience. Thank you for coming over at such short notice. Thank you for moving the table. Thank you for your support.

A note on compliments

'Really? I've had it ages.' 'You should see what he's like at bedtime.' 'I don't feel radiant, it's all make-up.' We reject compliments because we feel unworthy of the kind words. If the words don't match up to how we feel about ourselves, we reject them. It's the same reason why 70 per cent of lottery winners lose it all within three years and are three-to-five times more likely than the average adult to declare bankruptcy.[48] If we don't believe we're worthy of something, we'll consciously or subconsciously sabotage it.

Learn to accept compliments. Say 'thank you'. I know we've been trained to be self-deprecating, not to get too big for our boots, to stay small, but we're mothers now and we don't want that to trickle to the next generation, so say 'thank you'. A client once came to me desperate for more appreciation from her partner and children. 'I feel ignored and undervalued,' she said. I asked her about accepting compliments. She looked confused. If you want to feel more appreciated, the first step is to learn to accept the appreciation you're already getting. Then we worked on how she was going to feel more appreciation from her family.

Confident decision making

My client Donna told me: 'I want to be able to make quick and confident decisions, without hours of research, double guessing myself, finally making a decision, and then overthinking about it for weeks afterwards.' A 2022 Noom study found that adults make, on average, 122 decisions a day and that we change our mind twice for every decision.[49] I suspect the number is higher for parents and increases depending on the number of children you have. I used to be terrible at decisions and it impacted every area of my life, from the important to the every day. I was the person in the restaurant who'd order, then change my order five minutes later, then get food envy and wish I'd ordered differently. If this unimportant decision kicked me into overthinking, can you imagine how hard I found it to make important decisions?

I realized early on in my matrescence that my decision-making abilities needed a significant upgrade. I didn't have the time or energy for my usual overthinking, mind-changing habits, and unconfident decision making. The number of decisions I was having to make doubled now I was responsible for another human, and my time halved. I needed to find a way to make quick, confident decisions. I studied decision making, read books and studies, and tested out so many different tools and approaches to come up with the tool I'm about to teach you.

Decision-making toolkit

1. How important is it?

We have to be able to quickly assess how important a decision is, to give the right amount of time and energy to it. Decision fatigue is the psychological term when you have made too many decisions in a day, and you might be unable to make a decision or else feel overwhelmed by it. This is why a simple question at the end of the day ('What's for dinner, Mum?' or 'What do you want for dinner?') can send us over the edge (while staring at the open fridge door silently crying). We only have so much decision-making capacity, so when our days are full of micro decisions, we can lose the motivation for bigger, more important ones, such as: should we change schools? Do I need a new job? Are we happy living in this area? Decision fatigue can mean we avoid making big decisions altogether, letting others decide for us, or we continually procrastinate.

The real kicker with these more important decisions is that our brains crave certainty – we want to know we're making the right decision, but it's impossible to know with absolute certainty whether a decision is the right one or not. But this is hard to accept, especially when it comes to impacting our children. So, we ask too many people, do too much research, overthink and overworry, or maybe just ignore the issue altogether. When I asked my client Donna about her decision making, she told me it was the shame of getting it wrong that paralysed her: 'I come from a family where the need to be "right" ruled. I was laughed at and criticized when I got something wrong.'

If you were mocked or criticized when growing up for getting it 'wrong', then it makes complete sense that you put pressure on yourself to get it 'right' in adulthood. Much of our academic system focuses on getting the right answers, in the right ways. And as our brains are growing and forming up until the age of twenty-five, this will have had an impact on our fear of getting it 'wrong' for life. But we can brace ourselves for criticism, both from ourselves and others, when making a decision. The key is to take the pressure off your decision making.

Motherkind Toolkit: How important is this decision?
The next time you are faced with making a decision, give it a rating from zero to ten, where zero is unimportant and ten is very important. Ask yourself, will this matter in a week? A month? Next year?

If the decision rates as five or under, make the decision quickly and move on. If it's a five or over, follow the process below.

2. Ask yourself before asking others

My client had a decision to make about moving jobs. She was a single parent who loved her work as a doctor in a busy central-London hospital, but she wanted to be closer to her family for childcare support when her daughter started school and wanted a quieter life. She had spent a lot of time ruminating and thinking about her options and as I asked her to talk me through them, I saw how she was seeing the negative in each option because she was imagining how people in her life would judge her for her choices. I asked my three magic questions for cutting through the noise of others' expectations to get back to your truth:

1. What would I do if I knew I couldn't get it wrong?
2. What would I do if I knew I wouldn't be judged?
3. What would I do if I stepped into my most confident, powerful self?

She answered each one quickly and easily, as is often the case when we give ourselves permission to think about a decision with freedom from the weight of expectations, pressures, and judgement. In just sixty minutes together she went from confused and overwhelmed to knowing exactly what she wanted to do.

Asking others and doing research is an important part of decision making, but it's vital to consider your own opinions first. As women we're used to running our actions through the lens of others' needs, so this might be uncomfortable at first. I'm not suggesting we ignore others' needs or opinions, just that we check in with ourselves first. It might be that we know exactly what we want to happen, but it's not possible because of the needs of a co-parent, a legal agreement, or a practical need like school or nursery, but knowing what we want to do is an important muscle to develop, even if we then have to compromise on the actual actions we take.

Creative mentoring

Dr Tara Swart, neuroscientist and author of *The Source*, told me about an incredible decision-making tool called Creative Mentoring, which uses physical movement and therefore engages a different part of your brain.

1. Pose a problem you're facing now as a question. Take seven steps backwards and imagine yourself seven years ago. Say out loud how old you were seven years ago and what you were doing. Ask the younger you to give yourself advice about the question.
2. Come back to the centre. Take seven steps forward and imagine yourself seven years into the future. State how old you will be and ask the future you to give you advice about the question.

This simple tool is quick but incredibly powerful because it brings perspective into the decision-making process while drawing on the wisdom of our past selves and the dreams of our future selves.

3. Don't ask someone who hasn't been there

One of my favourite podcasts is *We Can Do Hard Things* with Glennon Doyle. At the end there's a line in the closing song which my brain takes a highlighter to every time I hear it: 'Stop asking people for directions to places they've never been.' Asking other people for advice is complex: most people will answer from their own experience, because what else do they have to draw on? Clinical psychologist Dr Nicole LePera believes that people give advice to their younger selves, not the person in front of them. When my best friend asked my advice about moving to Barcelona, I found it so hard to prevent my grief at her not living in the same city as me from impacting my thoughts.

Don't ask for your friend's opinion on leaving your job to set up your passion project if she's been stuck in a job she hates for ten years. Don't ask your parents about whether you should leave your unhappy marriage if they're unhappily married. The more people you ask, the more conflicting opinions you will get. The more opinions you collect, the further you'll feel from your own truth. It's like when you're scrabbling around for your keys; the more stuff piled on top of them, the harder they are to grab. Listening to yourself first is your key – don't pile so many opinions on top of your keys that you can't find them anymore. The golden rule is this: does this person have what I want in this area? Find someone – this could even be someone you don't know that well, such as a friend of a friend – who has experience in the area you're making the decision in and ask them.

I do several quick internet searches every day: what is the best way to get stains out of a white shirt? What time is that television show on tonight? When do the school holidays start? (Why have I still not printed the term dates and stuck them on the fridge? See page 91 for more on the mental load and why those small tasks still haven't been done.) The internet is an incredible resource and I'm grateful for it every day, but there's a big difference between asking for facts and information over asking strangers on the internet what we should do with this one wild and precious life. Glennon Doyle told me, 'I knew I'd hit rock bottom when I googled: what should I do if my husband is a cheater but also an amazing dad? I've just asked the *internet* to make the most important and personal decision of my life. Why do I trust everyone else on Earth more than I trust myself?'

Be mindful of what is productive research, i.e. acquiring knowledge needed to make the decision, versus unproductive research, i.e. procrastinating. Ask yourself, are you looking for an answer that doesn't exist?

We also need to be mindful of not giving unsolicited advice to others. My rule is this: unless someone specifically asks for my advice, I don't give it. Most people don't really want advice, they want to be heard. When we give advice, we want to fix. It feels controlling, because it is. If someone asks you directly, go for it. If not, try only to validate, hear, and hold their experience.

4. Accept imperfect decisions

After the pandemic we made the big decision to move from the city to the coast. We knew no one, had no family or friends close by, but we had a hunch that raising our girls by the sea would be beautiful. But when it came to making the leap, I was paralysed. What if we didn't like it? What if the girls didn't get on at school? What if we didn't make any friends? I was stuck in the worry spin discussed on page 274. Then Guy, my husband, set me free: 'Is the coast better than where we are now?' he asked me. 'Yes, definitely,' I said. 'So, we don't need to make the perfect decision,' he said. 'Just one that moves us forward into what we think will make us happier.' We moved the following month, and it was definitely the right decision.

You can't make the perfect decision because it doesn't exist. What we can do is make the best decision we can, based on our current knowledge and circumstances. Not many decisions are irreversible, and every decision we make about our own and our children's lives will give us information we can use to make better or different decisions in future.

> **Motherkind Moment**
> There are no perfect decisions, just choices we make to the best of our ability with the knowledge we have at the time.

It's far more painful not to make a decision – to procrastinate, over-think, and ruminate – than it is to make one, learn, and do it all over again. Action brings more clarity than thinking, researching, and procrastinating ever will.

A note on judgement

Judgement is in the air we breathe, so we need to build a filter.

Motherhood is one of the roles in society that is judged the most, but I don't need to tell you that, do I? Judgement of mothers is in the air we breathe; we're judged for every decision we make and often by those who are supposed to love and support us the most. We're judged for our parenting, our choices, how our children sleep, what we feed them, what they wear, the names we choose, the schooling we choose, where we choose to live, our bodies, and our work. We're judged for screen time, mealtimes – in fact all the time.

Every choice we make will be judged by someone, and the quicker we can accept that, the quicker we'll feel freedom from the fear of judgement, because it impacts our confidence more than anything else. Judgement won't ever stop; it is ingrained in motherhood, so we have to learn to become immune to it.

Don't let judgement change you

My friend was breastfeeding her four-year-old in a restaurant, and I thought, 'That's too old to breastfeed, especially in public. What will people think?' I smiled as she fed but I was shocked at how much I was judging her. The moment I got home, I grabbed my journal and asked myself what this was bringing up in me. In about thirty seconds I realized what was happening: her ease and joy at feeding for four years was touching on my pain and insecurity at not being able to breastfeed for as long as I wanted. *I was judging because I felt insecure.* I was nervous about her being judged by others because I was so self-conscious when I tried to feed in public, and even though she was completely confident, I was projecting onto her. I realized that every time I judge someone else, I find it's a part of me that feels insecure. We judge others when we also judge ourselves.

Motherkind Moment
When people judge you it's not about you at all; it's about their own insecurities. Judgement is so high in motherhood because there is so much insecurity.

When your mother-in-law judges your choice, she is really projecting her insecurity onto you about her own choices. As discussed on page 206, we need to imagine a glass wall between us and those judging us and give their insecurities back to them. Do not let others' judgements impact your actions. Everyone has a right to their opinion, just as we have a right to ours, but that doesn't mean we should let those opinions and judgements knock us off course. Never let other people's opinions take your power as a mother away – as a friend once said to me, 'Don't let other people's opinions live rent free in your head.' Perhaps former First Lady Eleanor Roosevelt said it best: 'No one can make you feel inferior without your consent.'

Motherkind Musing
- Who do you feel judged by?
- How does it impact you?
- How would your motherhood change if you didn't listen to or fear the judgement of others?

When someone criticizes you

Let's be honest, it hurts to feel criticized. I am very sensitive to criticism, which when hosting a podcast is not an ideal quality, so I've had to learn how to handle criticism without spinning out into self-loathing. Here's what I've learned:

- We can be hypervigilant to criticism and may think someone else is judging or criticizing us when in fact they aren't.
- We can't control what people think of us, only what we think of ourselves.
- Criticism will sting the most in areas we already feel insecure, so we can use it to learn where we need to develop confidence.
- No one else knows what we're facing.
- Some people connect through criticism of us or others, often without even realizing it. When you notice this create a boundary for yourself.
- We don't owe anyone an explanation, unless we want to give one.

Spread kindness to a hundred mothers today

I want to see less judgement and more support in motherhood, and I'm sure you do too – so we can be the change we want to see. We can make it our mission to support and be kind to every mother who crosses our paths.

Scientists at Harvard and Yale studied the contagiousness of kindness. They found that if you are kind to someone, they are more likely to be kind to someone else. On average one act of kindness reaches five people, and those five people reach another five, until a single act of kindness has reached 125 people.[50] Kindness can build confidence both in ourselves and others. So, as well as having the courage to take action, we can also have the compassion to spread kindness.

If you only have five minutes today ...

- Almost every mother wants more confidence in herself but doesn't know how to develop it.
- Confidence is a skill; it isn't something we're born with.
- Confidence grows with experience. It can feel so elusive in motherhood because so much is new, at every age and stage, and with each child.
- Confidence builds through taking imperfect action.
- Confidence isn't the absence of doubt, it's doing something despite the doubt.
- Confidence is not the same as extroversion.
- Confidence is having the courage to do what feels right to you.
- A lack of confidence in motherhood isn't our fault; there are many systems designed to undermine our confidence, but we can take responsibility for growing our confidence.
- We build confidence by embracing fear, starting small, accepting the inevitable discomfort, and becoming aware of when our limiting beliefs are impacting our confidence.

- Growth mindset is the skill of realizing that all growth comes from making mistakes and learning from those mistakes.
- Apologizing and rejecting compliments are two common behaviours in motherhood that undermine our confidence.
- Confident decision making is a vital skill in motherhood, which we can learn through the tools on page 259.
- Judgement is so high in motherhood because there is so much insecurity. We tend to judge others in areas where we ourselves feel insecure and when others judge us; it is about them, not us.

Chapter Eleven: Past, present, and future

'As you focus on clearing your generational trauma, do not forget to claim your generational strengths.'

XAVIER DAGBA, COACH AND MENTOR

I had dreamed of this moment. My heart melted when I saw her little hand lift up to wave at me in the audience, but as the nursery play started, I found myself struggling to stay present to watch it. My phone vibrating in my bag was a constant reminder of the work that waited for me, my busy mind was darting from what was for dinner to weekend plans, to wondering if that other mum was ignoring my smile on purpose. I knew the theory about presence – *The Power of Now* by Ekhart Tolle is one of my favourite books of all time – but in motherhood I found it harder and harder to actually be there, in body *and* mind. I was planning, worrying, ruminating, mental list making, but rarely in the moment. And hundreds of mothers I've spoken to share this same experience, rushing through our days, getting it all done, then lying down at the end of the day and thinking, 'Was I actually there for any of that?' It's like when we drive somewhere familiar but we don't remember the journey.

There is so much conversation in the parenting space about being present with our children, and it sounds easy, doesn't it? Every day I see videos on social media telling me that I only have eighteen summers with my children, or how quickly it passes, or to enjoy every moment. And while they may be well meaning, these messages are misinformed at best, and damaging at worse. No one enjoys every moment of anything. My wedding day was one of the best days of my life and I didn't even enjoy every moment of that. No one is even *aware* of every moment, let alone able to enjoy it.

Motherkind Moment
Being present is a skill that takes time to develop.

'Mummy, I've hardly seen you today,' my little four-year-old said at one bedtime. 'What do you mean, darling? We've been together all day.' It was then I realized I'd been distracted all day, busily rushing around from job to job. We had a quick chat at lunch, then off to the shops, then to collect her sister, then into the post-school whirlwind.

Some evenings my husband and I flop on the sofa together, both staring at a big screen with little screens in our hands. There is presence, we are together, but we definitely aren't present with each other: there's no talking, no eye contact, no sharing how we feel or what's on our minds.

My breakthrough came when I realized that it's not about how much time we spend with our children, it's the *quality* of that time that matters. Being *present* is the skill of being fully there: totally focused on the moment we're in. *Presence* is when we're there in body, but not in mind. Everything changed for me when I learned this difference. I stopped worrying about the hours I was spending with my children and started focusing on how present I could be in the pockets of time we spent together.

It's not about how much time we spend with our children, it's the quality of that time that matters.

Even though being truly present is a difficult skill to learn, it's worth practising because it's in the present moment that we can find more joy, connection, and peace. Even for a few precious moments, it's worth it.

Motherkind Moment
What really matters is how much emotional connection we can charge our children up with when we are together.

Fifteen is the magic number

How about we throw out 'enjoy every moment' and replace it with 'be fully present for fifteen minutes a day'? Feels better, right? Psychotherapist and author of *15-Minute Parenting* Joanna Fortune told me, 'You can most definitely do good connection in fifteen uninterrupted minutes.'

Joanna shares in her book that the quickest way to being fully present and emotionally connected with our children is through play. So, I started setting a fifteen-minute timer on my phone, asking the girls what they wanted to play, and going all in for fifteen minutes. Initially I found it hard to stay there in body and mind. My mind was wandering off to emails, podcast episodes, dinner plans, and missed calls. Every time I had a thought that wasn't focused on the play, I would practise letting it pass and think, 'Right now I'm playing,' and come back to the moment. It felt like a meditation practice (which is the practice of coming back to the present moment repeatedly). Children know when we are fully present with them and my girls loved it, and I could feel the emotional connection building as we'd giggle, do silly accents, and roll out the modelling clay. It's not the hours that count, it's how present you are when you're with your children.

But I'm addicted to my phone

I am, without a doubt, addicted to my phone. Selina Barker, author of *Burnt Out*, told me, 'When you think you've got a message, because you felt a vibration, and you look at your phone, and there isn't one, that is a sign of smartphone addiction. If you panic when you pop to the shops and you haven't taken your phone, and if you wake up in the morning, the first thing you do is you look at your phone and it's probably the last thing you do at night. These are signs of phone addiction.' We have to remember that we're the first generation of mothers holding everything we do while also holding onto a phone. And I'm not alone; 84 per cent of people worldwide said they couldn't go a day without their phone.[51]

In his 2017 TED talk, psychologist and screen expert Adam Alter said that the challenge with smartphones and social media is there is no 'stopping cue'. A stopping cue is a signal to move to another task and it used to be in all our media: a television show would end, the channel would stop broadcasting overnight, you would get to the end of the newspaper or magazine, but with smartphones there are no stopping cues, it just keeps going and going. Adam argues we have to create our own stopping cues and his is no phone while he's eating. Mine is no phone when I'm playing with the girls; it goes in a kitchen drawer when I make time for my fifteen minutes of present play with them. It's really hard and I notice my mind pulling me back to Instagram or WhatsApp. But I don't go and get my phone because with every behaviour you are either reinforcing a habit or breaking one.

I have worked hard on boundaries around work time and

non-work time with my phone. Every day I pick the kids up from school and this is time when I am not working. I say to myself, 'I am not working right now.' So, I don't answer work calls or emails, so I can be really present with them. But it wasn't always this way. I realized I had worked hard to squeeze my job into school hours so I could be with them after school, but I was spending that time on my phone, working. I was not present replying to emails and was not present with the girls: it was lose-lose. So, I decided that from pick-up time to bedtime was a no-work zone and it made a huge difference to our relationships.

Motherkind Musing

- How do you feel about your relationship with your phone?
- Are there any changes you need to make?
- What will you commit to?

The truth about worry

From the Motherkind community:
'I knew I was hugely missing out on connection with my children, my husband, and myself. Constantly projecting ahead in anxiety and worst-case scenarios or overthinking everything from the past. I was never really in the moment.'

Worry has robbed hours of joy from my motherhood. I would hate to add up the hours I have spent obsessing over worst-case scenarios that never happened. I have been a worrier my whole life, and in motherhood it increased massively. I have catastrophic thinking that projects the absolute worst case into a future that hasn't happened yet. When my husband is late or doesn't answer the phone,

I convince myself he's had a car accident. When my best friend says she needs to urgently speak to me, I decide that she's going to end our friendship forever. When one of my girls has a rash, I immediately grab a glass, convinced its meningitis. A Harvard University study showed we spend nearly half our waking life on autopilot, thinking about something other than what we are doing.[52] And I know for me, a lot of that thinking is worry.

But here's the thing: we worry so much because we *care* so much. We rarely worry about what we don't care about. In fact, the more we love someone, the more we worry. So, it makes sense that when it comes to our children, the worry increases to a whole new level.

I've had to find a way to hack my worried mind because after becoming a mother, it went into overdrive. And it doesn't get necessarily easier as our children get older; mothers of teenagers have told me that they worry more than ever. So, this skill of changing our relationship with worry is going to help us for *decades*.

Motherkind Moment
Today I will remember that my worry is a sign of how much I love.

Don't worry less, worry smarter

Years ago, when my mum was unwell, I worried non-stop about her. One day I was driving along so consumed with worry, I was so stressed and exhausted running through scenarios and 'what ifs' in my mind, that I nearly crashed the car. It was the wake-up call I needed – how devastated would my mum have been if I'd hurt myself? She didn't want me worrying, and it helped no one. I thought that by worrying I could somehow stop the worst from happening or that by worrying I would be better prepared if something did happen. Neither of which are true. I realized that because I felt so powerless and out of control, my worry felt like something I *could* do.

But worry doesn't help because it doesn't actually change anything, action does. It's like a car driving round in circles, using a lot of fuel and keeping busy, but not actually going anywhere. We need to give our worries a direction. We need to learn to differentiate between *productive* and *unproductive* worry.

Motherkind Moment

Productive worry is when our worry prompts actions that move us positively forwards. Unproductive worry is when our minds create problems that don't exist.

Yesterday I was worried I'd missed an important school deadline, so I checked and realized I had. I emailed the school office, and it was quickly sorted out. This worry was productive because it was a problem I could quickly solve. It didn't spin into overthinking and worst-case scenarios. But when I project a decade into the future and start worrying about the mental health of my girls, I am in unproductive worry, because there is no action, I can take today to solve that worry.

Motherkind Toolkit: Productive and unproductive worry

Think about a worry you have and ask yourself the following questions:

- Is this a problem I can solve?
- Am I in control of this problem?
- Is this a problem in the present?
- Can I start to take action in the next week?

If you answered yes to all, jot down the first action you need to take. If you answered no to any of these questions, then this is an unproductive worry.

Our thoughts are like wild horses, galloping worst-case thoughts through our minds. In order to find more peace of mind we need to learn to let the horses gallop past, not saddle up and jump on for the ride. We can do this by becoming aware of the thoughts. The moment we are aware, we have given ourselves a choice whether to saddle up or not. We can say to ourselves, 'I am worrying about something that hasn't happened.' It's like pressing pause; it doesn't mean the thoughts stop, but it makes it easier not to get carried away with them.

Motherkind Moment
If I am worrying about something that hasn't happened and likely never will, I can say to myself, 'This isn't today's worry.'

We never worry about the best-case scenario, do we? We become directors of a movie in the future, where the worst happens to all the actors. We press fast forward in our minds, quickly flicking through ten scenes to a bad ending. But things are rarely as bad as we worry they might be. I bet you can think of something you were really worried about – maybe a new job, or going back to work after maternity leave, or settling your child into a new nursery. I bet it wasn't as bad as your mind would have had you believe.

When we reflect on our past worries, we realize the common is far more likely to happen than the catastrophic. What if we gave equal weight to what we want to happen? Isn't it funny how much headspace we give to what we don't want to happen and how little we give to what we *do* want?

> **Motherkind Musing**
> What is the best that might happen?

> **Motherkind Toolkit: Tame worry**
> Practise reframing your thinking from the 'what ifs' to the 'what is'. Keep coming back to your current reality.

We worry when we think we can't handle the future. But we have handled every single challenge that has come our way up to this point in our lives, so why would the future be any different? We have mental files of evidence that we can do hard things, and we need to remember our strength when our minds worry about our inability to cope in a future worst-case scenario.

When the curveballs come

Curveballs come thick and fast in motherhood, don't they? We think if we organize enough, colour code, make lists, plan meticulously, then everything will be under control. But this is an illusion, and the truth is, we can't control the curveballs. An unwell child, a sick family member, an affair, an unwanted house move, a pandemic, financial challenges – the list is endless. The global pandemic curveball taught many of us that accepting what happens is more of a useful skill than trying to control what doesn't.

Motherkind Moment

The quicker you can accept what is happening, the quicker you can take action where you do have some control.

Accepting doesn't mean it's okay or that we're happy about what has happened. It means we accept our current reality as reality, and we stop wasting energy fighting it. It has happened, now what do we do? One of my favourite spiritual teachers, Ekhart Tolle, once said in a talk at the Albert Hall, 'Stress is caused by being "here" but wanting to be "there", and that is an incredibly useful idea for handling motherhood's curveballs.

Motherkind Toolkit: Accept, Prioritize, Trust

Accept where you are now. Resisting takes energy you don't have.
Prioritize what you need to do right now. What is your capacity? How have your priorities changed?
Trust in your ability to handle the curveball – you have handled every single one up to this point in your life.

Therapist and author Sandy C. Newbigging told me this powerful fable, and I remember it whenever I'm spiralling with worry about the curveballs.

A farmer and his son had a beloved horse who helped the family earn a living. One day, the horse ran away and their neighbours exclaimed, 'Your horse ran away, what terrible luck!' The farmer replied, 'Good or bad, who knows?' A few days later the horse returned home, leading a few wild horses back to the farm as well. The neighbours shouted out, 'Your horse has returned, and brought several horses home with him. What great luck!' The farmer replied, 'Good or bad, who knows?' Later that week, the farmer's son was trying to ride one of the horses when it threw him to the ground, breaking his leg. The neighbours cried, 'Your son broke his leg, what terrible luck!' The farmer replied, 'Good or bad, who knows?' A few weeks later, soldiers from the national army marched through the town, recruiting boys for the army. They did not take the farmer's son, because he had a broken leg. The neighbours shouted, 'Your boy is spared, what tremendous luck!' To which the farmer replied, 'Good or bad, who knows? We'll see.'

The paradox we need to embrace

I worry so much about my children facing pain. I worry that they'll be bullied, feel the sting of rejection if they're not chosen for the sports team, or feel lonely if they struggle to make friends. I worry that they'll be heartbroken by their first love or won't find love. What I forget is that I have grown and changed the most through facing these challenges. I wouldn't have wished for some of the things I've been through, but without a doubt the challenges have developed qualities in me that lay dormant before. I would never want to go through the challenges again AND I'm grateful for the depths they helped me find in myself. Both are true. Going through hard things *is* what makes us resilient.

> **Motherkind Moment**
> We develop resilience by facing life's challenges, and our children are no different.

Pain has gifted me with more wisdom than joy ever has – my friend and therapist Donna Lancaster calls this 'a present with a turd-shaped bow'. Heartbreak has made me more compassionate and softer. A suicide in my family has made me revere the preciousness of life. A loved one's mental health challenges has helped me learn how to hold boundaries and protect myself while opening my heart to someone else's pain at the exact same time. Unbelievable pain *and* beautiful lessons. Both are true.

Yet, I don't want my children to go through any pain. So much of my unproductive worry would pass if I could just accept that they *will* go through pain. And maybe, just like me (and probably like you), they will get through it. Maybe they'll even grow from it. This is the paradox we need to embrace: I don't want my children to face any hard times, but I know that's how they'll grow.

Dr Shefali, author of *The Conscious Parent*, told me, 'All of us are going to have pain. All of us are going to be heartbroken. Every one of us is going to experience failure, everyone is going to not be liked, not be the most popular. This is part of life ... I understand that, no matter what I do in my own life, I cannot avoid pain ... that no matter what I do in my child's life, I cannot avoid her pain. So why even try to avoid what's inevitable? The best thing I can do is to be there when I fall, I can be there for myself and be there when my kid falls, and to teach them that this is part of life. Pain is unavoidable.' What if instead of worrying about the inevitable pain our children will face, we could trust that those thorny bushes they will walk through will make them scratch-proof?

Motherkind Community: Sarah's story

My client Sarah described her struggles with presence to me when we first met. She had been struggling in the background for years, but motherhood magnified these difficulties. She described that becoming a mum was the only thing she felt certain about, an identity she loved, but it also left her feeling lost.

> 'I knew I was hugely missing out on connection with my children, my husband, and myself. I was constantly projecting ahead in anxiety and worst-case scenarios, or overthinking everything from the past, and never really in the moment'.

Struggling with a fierce inner critic, Sarah was exhausted from being constantly switched on to everyone around her and scanning for information that would inform her every move. It would take her ages to switch off after social events as she analysed whether she was 'good enough', or if that critic in her head was correct. She felt inauthentic and frustrated with herself. Like so many of us, Sarah would use social media and television to either numb her feelings or seek a connection. When we first began working together, Sarah found it difficult to name her emotions or her needs. What helped Sarah was reconnecting to her values and her strengths.

> 'I still remember this incredible feeling of lightness when I was able to see how these adapted behaviours, which I thought were my permanent personality traits, were coping mechanisms I had lovingly and cleverly formed to help protect myself and achieve the accomplishments I did as a child and adult. I felt I could begin to strip off the armour I had created, find the real me again, and accept my imperfections. Now my intuition is so important to me. I follow my inner wisdom of what feels best for myself and my family. This then naturally ensures I honour my values and my authenticity. I provide my own validation and am much more present and connected with my family. We discuss our needs and feelings and encourage the boys to tune into their intuition. We discuss their strengths and encourage them to validate themselves for their achievements. This is what I want for my lovely boys'.

Why our past keeps knocking on the door of the present

One day my daughter came home and told me she'd spent lunchtime sitting on a bench alone because no one wanted to play with her. She was quite happily telling me this, seemingly unbothered, but I could feel the emotion rising in me and I wanted to burst into tears. I managed to hold it together and chat to her about how she felt, but later that evening I still couldn't stop thinking about it. How rejected she must have felt, how lonely, how unpopular and unloved. I burst into tears.

Then I realized it wasn't her I was crying about, it was me.

I remembered I'd had exactly the same experience when I was the same age, but had totally forgotten about it until that moment, and the unprocessed emotion of my little five-year-old self came flooding back. I let my tears flow and told myself exactly what I needed to hear back then: 'There is nothing wrong with you, everyone gets left out sometimes, you are loved.' This is called 'reparenting', when we give ourselves in the present what we needed in the past, and I'll dive into it shortly.

> **Motherkind Moment**
> I had no idea how much I'd be reminded of my own little self when I was raising little selves.

I have released over seventy podcast episodes on how our past impacts our present, because I feel passionately that this needs to be talked about more. I had no idea, blissfully rubbing my belly, that my skill set in motherhood would need to include being able to work out how my past was still impacting me today. And I'll bet you didn't either. But it's totally normal, and even world-leading parenting expert Dr Shefali told me: 'I was shocked to find how much unresolved stuff I had.' So, it's a vital skill to develop, because it will enable us to create a version of motherhood on our terms, free from whatever might have happened in our past.

Just like with my daughter's playground experience, when you have a disproportionate reaction to something, it's a nudge telling you that it's touching on something from your past that still hurts. Perhaps if your child had told you of a different experience to your own, it wouldn't have impacted you at all, because it wouldn't have pushed on one of your painful memories. Psychotherapist Philippa Perry told me, 'If in response to your child, you get a very charged emotion, then that is a hint and a clue that that charge belongs in the past and not the present.'

When our jaw locks when our child has a public meltdown, or when we feel our chest constricting when our toddler says 'no' to us, or we burst into tears when our child is left out, this is useful information telling us about where we might have a past pain that is coming back in the present. Dr Rangan Chatterjee, author of *Happy Mind, Happy Life*, told me, 'It's not because [my children] have done something, it's because it's triggered something in my past that I have not resolved.'

And it goes even deeper …

We will be most reactive to experiences that happened to us at the same age as our children are now. I was five when I had the experience of feeling left out, so it's not surprising that it was when my five-year-old told me about the same experience that I had a big emotional reaction. I suspect if she'd been older or younger, it might not have affected me in the same way. But because I knew what was happening, and I felt able to hold myself through it, a little part of me grew stronger that day. I had forgotten about that seemingly small but clearly important experience and it was my reaction to my daughter that meant it could bubble up to the surface, so I could deal with it and move on.

Unpleasant and frustrating as it is to be knocked sideways by past experiences when we're just trying to get on with juggling everything in our lives, I have come to learn it can actually be positive. This is because every time we process one of these triggers, we grow in self-awareness and heal a part of ourselves at the same time.

I realized how significant that playground experience was for me by how big my reaction was to my daughter, and when I thought about it more deeply, I still had the belief that I wasn't liked (which we discussed in Chapter Two). So that memory resurfacing gifted me the chance to rewrite history and replace it with a new belief – 'I am loved' – then look for evidence that this is true (following the beliefs process on page 41). Psychotherapist Louis Weinstock agreed when he told me: 'When your child gets to a certain age, where you have some unresolved wound, your child is designed to trigger you in a particular way. It's almost like life is giving you a chance to heal this thing that you haven't healed, if you are open enough to take it.' We can reframe these memories and triggers from a frustration to a gift because we are being given the opportunity to heal what happened to us. And perhaps one day, when we look back, we might even be grateful.

Motherkind Toolkit: The six whats

Next time you have a reaction to someone or something (it could be your children, friend, partner, stranger in the supermarket) ask yourself:
- What am I feeling about this situation?
- What does this remind me of?
- What story or belief about myself is this bringing up?
- What age does this feeling remind me of?
- What words do I need to say to myself now that I didn't have then?
- What do I need to do now?

Doing this exercise will help you work through any emotional reaction, big or small. But be sure to do it imperfectly – you might not have any answers for some of the questions and that's more than okay. Remember the 1 per cent rule: even a small amount of new self-awareness will help you feel more confident and empowered in your ability to handle the many challenges you face. If anything comes up for you that you feel unable to handle on your own, please seek professional support.

You can give yourself now what you needed then

What is so incredible about this curiosity-led approach is that we can give ourselves now what we needed when we were younger, and it still counts. The cliché that it's never too late to have a happy childhood is true because we can make up for whatever we might have needed or wanted then, now. So, if you needed more affection and love, you can give that to yourself now, or ask others for more. If you wanted more fun, you can have more fun now. If you wanted more play, you can play more now. If you wanted to be truly seen for who you are, you can give that to yourself now. You can fully love, accept, and see yourself now. What a gift.

Sometimes I joke that I have three children: my two girls and my own little self (my inner child) because I find it so joyful and healing to watch my children grow and at the same time think about giving my younger self whatever she might have needed but didn't get. So, as I mother my girls with as much compassion, kindness, presence, and understanding as I can muster, I am also giving all those gifts to myself. As our children remind us of what happened to us, we can ask ourselves how we wish our own caregivers had handled situations and ask ourselves if we can give ourselves that now.

If you were criticized for making a mistake when you were younger, and it didn't feel great, you can now respond to yourself with kindness and compassion when you make a mistake. If harsh words were used, you can use kind words with yourself. If you were bullied, you can give yourself love. What a beautiful miracle it is to be parenting ourselves alongside our children. By doing this we become cycle breakers.

Motherkind Moment
A cycle breaker is someone who intentionally wants to create a different pattern of behaviour than they were taught growing up.

We are all cycle breakers, because every single one of us wants to do at least one thing differently than we experienced growing up. Even if you had the most incredible childhood, there will still be some things you want to change as you create your own family. We're the brave ones, standing at a crossroads, looking at the old, well-trodden path of how generations of our families did things and choosing another path, a road less travelled, like fresh snow with no footprints. Maybe there's lots of cycles you want to break, maybe just a few, but you're the one standing there holding your child's hand saying: 'Let's create a new story.' You're the one doing the courageous, hard work of doing it differently. Perhaps you're the first mother in your family to go to therapy, to stop drinking, to do motherhood alone, to work, to not work, or to know your worth. Maybe you're the first mother down your lineage who says enough to the pain passed down the generations like a baton in a relay. Maybe you're determined to be the first mother to truly believe and value herself, to go for your dreams and see what you're capable of. Maybe you want to be the first to accept and love her body, free from diets and self-loathing. Maybe you want to be the first to not punish, hit, or shame your child. Maybe you want to create a family based on kisses, cuddles, and love, not fear and criticism. Even when your choices might be judged and shamed, you know that there is a different way and I want you to honour yourself now for how incredible you are.

> **Motherkind Moment**
> The family you came from doesn't need to define the family that comes from you.

'I'm the First Lady of the United States but my greatest challenge is rais-ing two girls more compassionate and wise than the generation before.'
MICHELLE OBAMA

I believe every generation wants to do better than the one before. The greatest gift we can give to our children is what we ourselves were never given.

But how do we actually do it? How do we gather all the amazing lessons and qualities we've learned from our own lives and make sure we pass them on? And how do we leave what we don't want to repeat in the past where it belongs? It all starts with awareness. Imagine you're in a ball pit at a soft-play centre and everywhere you look there are different-coloured balls – you're swimming in them. I'm going to show you how to organize them into two buckets, which are credits (what I want to repeat) and debits (things I want to change).

Motherkind Toolkit: Debits and credits

Without awareness, we risk unconsciously repeating or rejecting what we saw or were taught in childhood, so this coaching tool is like pausing for a moment to take stock. I believe it's one of the most empowering things we can do because just as an entrepreneur has to look at her balance sheet to get clarity about her business, we too have to look at our own personal balance sheet to get the awareness and clarity so we can move forward with more freedom from the past.

Complete the below table for your debits and credits; you can use the categories and prompts on page 290 to help you. It's up to you how deep you go with this, and you can return to it many times – each time you'll learn something new about yourself. As you move through your motherhood journey, new awareness will come to you at each age and stage, so I encourage you to return to this tool whenever you need to.

Trust that whatever you write down will be exactly what you're meant to – try not to control this or do it perfectly remember that even 1 per cent more insight and awareness will be powerful. This exercise isn't about right or wrong or blame – it's about awareness, like turning the light on in a dark room, and once completed, we'll be able to see much more clearly where we're going.

Credits	Debits
What have I learned in my life so far that I want to pass on?	What do I want to do differently?

Emotional support

When something bad or sad happened, did you feel emotionally supported? What were you taught about feelings and emotions? Was your emotional self validated and encouraged? What have you learned about emotions you want to pass on?

Expectations

What were your parents' expectations of you? How were you encouraged to behave? What were the expectations of the mothers in your family? What did you see modelled about motherhood? What are your expectations of yourself as a mother?

Values

What was valued in your childhood? What was important in your family? How was that shown? Were your own values respected? What values do you want to instil in your family?

Relationships

What was modelled to you around relationships? How was love shown, to you and the other adults? What did you learn about relationships? What have you learned about relationships in your adult life?

Worth

How was self-worth modelled to you? Who had the most worth in your family? The least? What were you taught about self-worth? What have you learned about self-worth through your life?

Now that you're aware of your debits and credits, you can use this new awareness to make changes.

1. Reflect

What did you learn from the debits and credits? How did they impact you and form you into the person you are today?

2. Repeat

How can you ensure that you repeat the credits? What rituals, traditions and values do you need to make sure you bring into your family?

3. Reparent

How can you give yourself what you weren't given? What might you need to learn? How can you learn these new skills together with your children?

4. Remove

What patterns do you want to leave in the past? How can you use the debits as positive fuel for creating your own family? What is a non-negotiable action, behaviour, or belief that you won't repeat?

Hopefully this exercise has given you a new perspective, self-awareness, and fuel for what you want to do differently. If you have a partner, co-parent, or caregivers, it's a fantastic exercise to discuss and do together. It's important to remember that it's inevitable we will pass on some of what we don't want to. I used to put myself under so much pressure to break every cycle I was aware of, and it was crippling. Now, I try my best, I stay aware of the credits I want to bring into my children's lives, and I do my best to counter my debits. But I do it imperfectly and so will you, because life is imperfect. This is absolutely not something to put yourself under pressure about, but let the gentle hand of awareness be your guide. Awareness is an incredible gift, because when I realize I'm stuck in perfectionism, or people pleasing, or pushing down my needs, I'm aware of it, and that gives me a choice. That is real freedom.

Doing this exercise and understanding the generational patterns in my family completely changed how I saw my relatives. Birthing my own daughters, I realized the enormity of the role and I connected for the first time with a deep sense of gratitude for everything my own parents gave me. Despite there being many debits on my list, the grace I extended to my own parents comes back to me too. The more I can accept the messy humanness of my parents, the more I'm able to accept my own.

One of signs that you're maturing emotionally is that you can see your parents or caregivers as flawed humans, trying the best they could with what they had. This isn't about letting someone 'off the hook' or saying that what happened was okay – far from it. But acceptance is giving up all hope of a different past. It means that we accept what happened, take the lessons, and move on to create a future on our own terms, and in doing so, we set ourselves free from the past.

If you only have five minutes today …
- Being present with our children and in our lives is a hard but important skill to develop.
- Being there (presence) is not the same as connecting (being present). We can practise being fully present with our children for just fifteen minutes a day.
- Phone addiction is a common challenge that stops us being present, so we have to put boundaries in place.
- Worry is massive in motherhood, because we care so deeply and our minds are wired to worry.
- We can learn to differentiate between productive and unproductive worry.
- Curveballs are when the unexpected happens and the Accept, Prioritize, Trust tool (see page 279) will help you to recover from any setbacks.
- We worry so much about our children facing any pain or challenge, but actually it's pain and challenge that helps each of us grow and develop qualities in ourselves.

- Our past keeps coming up in motherhood because our children remind us of what happened to us at the same age.
- Our 'inner child' can be activated by what we see our own children going through.
- Even though this is hard, it actually can help us heal old beliefs and patterns, because we can only change what we can see.
- We can use the Six Whats tool (see page 285) to uncover what is really happening when we feel triggered by our children.
- We can 'reparent' ourselves by giving ourselves now what we might have needed when we were younger.
- A cycle breaker is someone who wants to do at least one thing differently than they experienced growing up.
- The Debits and Credits tool (see page 289) is a simple way to define what you want to repeat from your family of origin, and what you want to change for the family you are creating.

Chapter Twelve: A vision for motherhood

'We have two lives, and the second begins when we realize we only have one.'

CONFUCIUS

Every single one of you holding these pages or hearing my words will be facing different challenges, but we all face one opportunity: to allow motherhood to lift us into the foreground of our own lives. For too long the expectation of mothers has been the opposite: to become shadows behind our children's light. But what if we can all shine?

I once knew a woman who looked perfect from the outside; she was beautiful, kind, and loving to everyone around her. She was a doting mother, ever present, always busy with cooking, cleaning, sorting, and doing. She made the lives of everyone around her easier – facilitating joy for everyone else, but accepting crumbs for herself. She picked up pieces, socks, and snacks. She was always smiling, never letting a crack show. She buried her pain and dreams deep inside like a jewel never to be found and poured all her love into her children, perhaps not realizing it was her who needed it the most.

At age fifty, with children packed off with saucepans and ring binders to university, the cracks of decades of people pleasing and perfectionism became a crevasse and she found herself in a dark hole – you can't outrun your feelings in the revealing stillness of an empty nest. Step by step, she bravely climbed out, sifting through the rubble of the past, and feeling decades of unfelt feelings. By setting boundaries for the first time, she started to value, respect, and believe in herself. She saw the woman she was capable of becoming. She started therapy, found her true passions, and starting truly living. She transformed. She saw what she was capable of when she believed in herself. She became incredibly successful in her new career, and at sixty even found herself on a television show.

That woman is my mother. And I could not be more proud of her. It has been the privilege of a lifetime to watch my mother become the leading role in her own life. It's a universal truth that we want the people we love most to also love *themselves*. My mother inspired me to follow my dreams, to face the past, to see my children as a reason to stand in the foreground of my own life, and not hide in their shadows. I have had two mothers, both the same woman: one running from herself in busyness and the lives of her children, and one empowered and happy. I don't need to tell you which version has inspired me the most, which one I have been closest to, and which one has helped me become the woman I am today.

The gift of perspective

I'm sitting on the sofa sobbing while breastfeeding my two-week-old daughter. Not because of the pain of her latch, not because every suckle makes me wince, but because I'm watching *This Is Us*, which is quite possibly the most beautiful show I've ever seen. It follows the life of triplets, and each episode is a kaleidoscope of the day-to-day struggles of life and the perspective of the bigger picture by showing the generations of the family and spanning a hundred years of family history.

I sob as I realize the overwhelming nothingness of sitting here on a cold December morning, and yet the whole of my life is in my arms. I cry for versions of me I couldn't love. I cry for how much

I love this little person I barely know yet. I think about how there are more stars in the sky than grains of sand in the world. And I look into her eyes and know, to her, I am the sky and the stars.

In the final episode, the mother, Rebecca, dies and as she walks back through her life along a train, she meets former versions of herself. She sees mistakes she's made, the gifts she's given her children, and how it was all exquisitely, perfectly imperfect. I think about me in a line standing with hundreds of women behind me, and hundreds in front. I think about my mum behind me and my nan behind her. I stand tall and strong, and I think about the little shoulders in front of me, my two girls. I think about their possible future children in front of them, and theirs in front of them. I see myself as part of a beautiful chain of women, our features, strengths, traumas all passed down. And I think about what I want to pass on. What will be my gift to my ancestors and to the future generations? This is a big question, and you might not want to think with a wide lens right now, and that's more than okay. But if you're feeling stirred or maybe emotional by this idea then I want to offer you a coaching tool I offer my clients when we're coming to the end of our partnership. It invites you to think about yourself as an eighty-year-old.

> **Motherkind Toolkit: Your eightieth birthday**
> Close your eyes if you feel comfortable doing so.
>
> Imagine it's your eightieth birthday and your grown-up children and perhaps grandchildren have gathered around you.
>
> You look into their eyes and feel more love pouring back at you than you have ever felt.
>
> Then your children make a speech, and it opens with 'I've learned so much from my mother. I've learned what really matters in this life, and she's been an example to me of …'

What do they say next?

What were the magic moments in your life?

What did you teach them?

What did you show them from how you lived your life?

What made your life so meaningful?

What did you create?

Who did you love?

What mattered to you?

Being true to you

Therapist Donna Lancaster told me on the podcast that there are two parts to our lives. Phase one is where we are more focused on validation from others, where we think that 'things' like shoes and handbags will make us happy, and we want to look good on the outside. We focus on fitting in, being accepted, and doing what we think we 'should'. We look for things outside of us to complete us. We tick societal boxes of what we've been told a good life is: good job, nice things, own home. Donna calls this 'outside-in living'. We value how things look to others over how we feel on the inside to us. So, we might find ourselves looking into our baby's eyes or up at the stars one night thinking, 'Is this all there is?' Dr Rangan Chatterjee, author of *Happy Mind, Happy Life*, told me, 'I've got everything, why do I still feel worthless? From the outside, I ticked off society's definition of success. But in the early part of my career, I still felt a deep void inside me, even with this external metric of success.'

Before motherhood, I was in phase one. I looked great and had a good job. From the outside my life was good, but inside I didn't like myself. I didn't feel any passion for my job, had no idea what really brought me joy, and life felt like an academic tick-box exercise, with every day a rung notched on the wrong ladder.

Many things can begin the shift into phase two: grief, divorce, redundancy, a house move. For me, it was my matrescence that moved me into phase two of my life. In this second phase we feel less focused on status and more motivated by the truth of who we are. We become less driven by what others think of us, and more by what we think of ourselves. We might ask, 'Who am I really?' or 'What really matters to me in this life?' We begin to uncover what makes us uniquely us and begin to celebrate ourselves. It isn't that we don't enjoy the shoes and the achievements and the job titles, it's just that we know it doesn't define us anymore.

The shift from phase one to phase two isn't driven by age, and some people never make the dive into the deeper waters of phase two. Author of *Untamed* Glennon Doyle told me, 'I think it took me forty years to figure out that all I really had to do was return to myself by trying to remember who I was before the world told me who to be.'

I realized nothing outside of me was going to make me truly happy, and that was my responsibility. Holding new life in my arms, it no longer felt like an option to continue hating myself, keeping myself small, doubting my every move, and overthinking my every word. How could I raise bold, brave, compassionate children when I was falling inwards on myself with fear and self-doubt? Looking into my children's eyes, I saw nothing but pure love and potential. What if I could see that when I looked into my own? Could I become the mother they deserved? Steady, confident, assured. How could I pass on my wisdom if I didn't believe I had any? Motherhood has made me refuse to ignore my true self: what I really love, what I'm really capable of, my dreams. It made me stop living for the outside world and invited me inwards, to peel away layer after layer of 'shoulds' and 'have tos', to find out who I really am and what I really want. And there's less time for bullshit now – my own and other people's.

Bronnie Ware, author of *The Top Five Regrets of the Dying*, has been with thousands of people as they took their last breaths. After a few years, she started to notice a pattern in the regrets people would express in the last days of their lives. The most common regret she heard was this: 'I wish I'd had the courage to live a life true to myself, not the life others expected of me.' I remember right before I started Motherkind, the fears going through my mind were 'What will my old corporate boss think?' 'Will everyone laugh at me?' 'What will my friends think?' 'What will strangers on the internet think?' Imagine if I'd listened to those shackles, stayed small, and crumbled under the fears of other people's expectations of me. Imagine if I'd pleased everyone around me, kept my head down, stuck to a safe job, not risked trying something new, not risked failure, and not risked looking like a fool. You wouldn't be reading this right now.

Motherkind Community: Helen's story

You might remember Helen from page 127, who, like many of us, had absorbed other people's values while growing up and lost that vital connection with herself. I find her story of being true to herself inspirational. While discovering her values, Helen began to think about her own wellbeing and the impact that had on her child. She found that the most profound change in her matrescence had nothing to do with how to be with her son and everything to do with her relationship with herself. Helen began to understand some of her early programming and why this mattered. She also learned to recognize when her nervous system was activated, how to regulate herself, and develop self-compassion. The cumulative effect was that she began to understand herself, trust her intuition, and reconnect with parts of herself that had been suppressed along the way.

'One of the automatic consequences of all this change was that I didn't need so much advice about how to parent. I began to trust that the answers were in my intuition and in the relationship between my son and myself. I learned that in moments of calm, I can look inwards and be the kind of mother that feels authentic to me – to be present, playful, compassionate, and have boundaries ... I wish that every mother was able to internalize the belief that being a model, not a martyr, is truly the best thing you can do for yourself and your children. If it seems selfish to you and you struggle to do it for yourself, then do it for your children. This journey has not been easy, it has definitely not been linear, and it will certainly be a life-long process. But I am so grateful for all the changes. For the first time in my adult life, I feel present, conscious, and have begun to reconnect with my creativity and the things that light me up.'

I am truly the most happy I have ever been. I know my worth, I know that all the outside successes I sometimes get wrapped up in (will anyone buy this book?) are nice, but they are fleeting feelings. Like a firework exploding brightly, they look impressive but when those achievements end, I know that I'm okay. I know what truly matters to me. I know that when I look back on this phase of my life, I'll feel proud for how I prioritized my time and energy. I have stopped wasting my precious time on this planet, at this time, with these children, doing things I don't want to do, to impress people I don't like, and spending money to try to find that elusive sense of freedom and peace, when it was inside me all along.

The gift of knowing what truly matters

'And every day, the world will drag you by the hand, yelling, "This is important! And this is important! And this is important! You need to worry about this! And this! And this!" And each day, it's up to you to yank your hand back, put it on your heart and say, "No, this is what's important."'

IAIN S. THOMAS, POET

I love these words because every single day I forget what is really important to me.

We started together with the 'should sham' on page 30 and hopefully, through the chapters, you have connected more and more with what really matters to you in motherhood. So now let's pull it all together and give you the gift of space to think about what you really want.

Our challenge is that in the rush of day-to-day life everything matters. It feels important to me to get to school on time, to get homework done, to get dinner on the table at the right time, to reply to that message, and to wash and iron that top I want to wear tomorrow. And those things of course are important; they're the sprinkles on top, but they're not the cake.

One of the greatest gifts of motherhood for me has been the exquisitely heart-breaking front-row seat it gives you to observe the passing of time. Year to year I might notice a few more wrinkles or an extra roll of skin in the mirror, but week by week I get to watch my children change. Words once mispronounced are suddenly said correctly. Wobbly legs are suddenly running away from me. Nervous, tear-fuelled drop-offs become run-ins without a glance back. Motherhood, if you allow it, gives you a new perspective on life. Like when my girls scoop up sand at the beach into their sieve and shake it to reveal the rocks and pebbles left behind. Motherhood is a sieve for what really matters to you.

Health coach and wellness speaker Georgie Crawford asked me, 'Are you on the dance floor or the balcony of life?' When you climb the stairs to the balcony and look down at your life, what do you see? Perhaps you see yourself rushing around looking after everyone but yourself. Do you seem exhausted and frustrated? Perhaps you see yourself laughing with friends or playing with your children. Are you just surviving? Let's press pause on the music for a moment, freeze frame everyone and everything on the dance floor, and ask yourself: what matters to me?

What's your purpose?

What an awful question. As if there's just one purpose. Before motherhood, I used to think about purpose as a grandiose, philosophical quest and when I found it, I would feel the self-acceptance, confidence, and peace I'd been seeking all along. Thinking about purpose like that is setting yourself up for failure. Now I see purpose very differently. I define it as spending time on what is important to me. So a better question is: how can I best use my time on something that feels important to me?

> **Motherkind Moment**
> Purpose isn't just one thing. It's about understanding what's important to you and investing your time there.

What matters to me is to work every day on believing in myself, trusting myself, being the best mother I can be, and being of service in the world through my work. That purpose is with me when I'm with my girls and it's with me when I'm supporting mothers. It's with me when I'm alone and when I'm with friends. Shifting to see your purpose as something you can connect with every day will motivate and inspire you even through the hardest of seasons. Finding purpose every day is such a gift, because when we're swimming in the sea of routines, school runs, mental load, work meetings, and laundry it can feel like we're rudderless. But having clarity on what's really important will give us a sense of meaning every single day.

My client Laurie had stopped paid work to raise her three young children and came to me because she felt continually guilty and conflicted that she wasn't earning and progressing in her career. 'I feel like I'm wasting all those years building my career. I just don't know what my purpose is,' she told me. We sat in silence for a few minutes, allowing the space between us to act as a door to a different possibility. 'What is the most important thing to you right now?' I asked her. 'Being with my children,' she said without hesitation. 'Maybe that's your purpose right now. Maybe your purpose is to be all in with your children. To be fully with them. And maybe your purpose after that will be to grow your career again.' She started crying. 'What are the tears about?' I asked. 'Relief,' she said. It was as if she needed permission to truly accept her purpose. Caregiving has been so devalued in our society that we cannot trust our inner voice to tell us that it's our purpose right now. We are raising the next generation; what could be more important than that? Each of us will have a different answer to the purpose question – it doesn't matter what you answer – what matters is that you ask yourself the question.

Motherkind Musing
What is most important in your life right now?

Permission to dream

Your wants matter, your dreams matter, and your desires matter. And don't you forget it. I will no longer let you hide in the shadows of your own life – you're too important for that. I know what it's like as a child to watch a parent finally start believing in themselves. It's incredible to watch someone start feeling about themselves the way you feel about them.

I was recently telling a friend how writing this book has been my dream come true. I have dreamt of being an author since I was five years old. Later, at bedtime, my eight-year-old said to me, 'Mummy' ... I braced myself for a request of water/a banana/more screen time but instead she said, 'I'm proud of you.' 'Why?' I asked. 'Because you're making your dreams come true.' I burst into tears when

I realized what I was showing her, and that motherhood doesn't have to mean the end of your dreams.

It can be the beginning.

If you only have five minutes today ...

- Motherhood is an opportunity to raise ourselves too.
- It's powerful to think about ourselves in the context of past and future generations and how we want to live through what is truly important to us.
- The eightieth-birthday exercise (see page 296) invites you to think about yourself with a long-term perspective, which will help you make decisions and prioritize your time today.
- Therapist Donna Lancaster teaches that there are two phases to life: one which is driven by what others think of us and what we think we 'should' do and one where we focus on what feels truly meaningful to us.
- Motherhood can invite you to think about what really matters to you and what values you want to pass on to your children. It can reconnect us to our true selves.
- Your purpose is simply going all in on what is important to you right now. Your purpose will change through the different seasons of life.
- Motherhood doesn't have to mean the end of you and your dreams – it can be the beginning.

Just one gift

I'm sitting on a slightly damp bench at the park watching my two girls on the swings, the sun is on my face, and I feel present as its gentle rays warm my cold cheeks. I'm watching their little legs swing up and down as their hair covers their smiling faces. Nothing special, just a morning at the swings. But it does feel special. There's no inner critic pressuring me to join in or move us on, or get home to sort out the mess that awaits. I don't feel guilty that I've left work undone to go out in the sunshine. There are a million things going on: work challenges, family dramas, illnesses, and grief. But they hover above my head, like birds circling a nest, and they don't consume me. I feel present.

I look up and see the rhythmic motion, back and forth, back and forth, and with every swing I can feel joy bubbling up inside me, and a smile comes over my face. I realize I feel peaceful. I know in the next moment it will be gone, and that's okay, such is life: back and forth, back and forth. This is the gift of Motherkind, of living these principles and using these tools. Today, I have my own back, I know how to be present, worry no longer consumes me, my time is used wisely, and I don't bow down to pressures and perfectionism. Despite my full plate, I feel full of energy. My boundaries are strong, I say no a lot, and I know who I am. I am no longer a victim of the memo passed to me about what a mother is and does. I am imperfectly becoming a model, not a martyr. When I inevitably swing back into fear, comparison, pressure, and guilt, I will know I have a choice about how long I stay there. I have tools. And now, so do you.

I look at my girls' faces, and I see joy, freedom, and delight. And I realize for the first time that it's in me too. I have freed myself from the binds of the 'shoulds' and the 'have tos'. I have accepted that motherhood might never be celebrated, or recognized, or supported how we so desperately know it needs to be. Because sitting at the swings today I choose to celebrate, recognize, and support myself. I will no longer collude in the undermining of the privilege of a lifetime: to be a mother. There is always going to be someone who doesn't see my worth, but today, it won't be me.

My greatest wish for my girls is that they always have their own backs. The world can throw cruel words their way and they will know, deep inside, that they are good enough just as they are, so the words may sting, but they won't stick. That they will never abandon themselves. That they will love themselves enough to walk away from a toxic relationship, leave a soul-sucking job, take risks, have meaningful friendships, wear whatever they like whatever their size, have the courage to say no, to choose themselves over and over again until they've created a life so beautiful that one day they wake up and can't believe it's real.

But if I *really* want this for my children, I have to give it to myself too. I have to show them what it looks like to really live, to choose myself, over and over again until I've created a life so beautiful that one day I wake up and can't believe it's real. In the words of Glennon Doyle, I have to become a 'model, not a martyr'.

The principles that I've shared with you have changed my motherhood, and my life. I am unrecognizable from the needless, resentful, exhausted, and self-critical mother I once was. I am indebted to the hundreds of wise minds, kind souls, and knowledgeable authorities who have not only enabled this shift in myself, but have allowed me to share what has changed me with you too.

'What's the one gift you'd give to all mothers in the world and why?' I have heard 412 answers to this question because I ask it at the end of every single *Motherkind* episode. I have heard answers that have made me laugh, made my heart break, and made me cry. I've heard self-love, a time-travel machine, a night in a hotel once a month, unshakeable confidence, freedom from guilt, safety, self-trust, self-belief, and, one of my favourites, a wife.

But the gift I'd most like to leave you with is a new blueprint for motherhood, and here are the directions:

We need to care deeply about ourselves.
We need to transform our inner critic into an inner friend.
We need to believe in ourselves, even when no one else does.
We need to believe in each other.
We need to see guilt for what it really is: a way to keep us small.
We need to recognize our power.
We need to model, not martyr.
We need to protect our time and energy like the precious jewels they are.
We need to say no to what is draining us.
We need to say yes to what is lifting us.
We need the courage to break cycles.
We need boundaries, lots of them.
We need to question the rules, break the rules, and make our own rules.

You need to know deep in your bones that you are enough, and you always have been, and always will be. I believe that once we are free from what no longer serves us, it's our duty to help others do the same. My deepest hope is that I have done that, in some small or big ways, for you with my words.

Gratitude

This book has been both the greatest challenge and biggest achievement of my working life. Cheesy as it sounds, writing these words to you has been a dream come true. I wrote the majority of the book during the school summer holidays (note to self: don't do this again), which meant I had to use every single one of the tools in this book every single day. If it weren't for me taking my own advice on self-compassion, rest, letting go of guilt, asking for help and setting boundaries, there's no way you'd be reading these words now. This book is the result of eight years of research, thousands of hours of coaching, and over 400 podcast interviews. It has been the privilege of my life to take what I have learned from the incredible experts, clients, and Motherkind community and turn it into what I hope has been a supportive resource for you.

Thank you to every listener of the *Motherkind* podcast: without you this book just wouldn't exist. Thank you for listening, sharing, and spreading the message of *Motherkind* far and wide. I never take it for granted that you choose *Motherkind* to be your companion in motherhood – thank you. Thank you to every guest who has given me their time, expertise, and wisdom on the podcast. A special thank you to the experts whose words and ideas I have included in the book – thank you for your support and permission. I really do stand on the shoulders of giants. Thank you to my clients who have allowed me to share your stories in these pages – I am so inspired by and grateful to you.

Motherkind is a team effort. Thank you to my team past and present for joining me on this mission. Jo, Angie, Kelly, Josie, and Nicola – thank you for your hard work and passion. I couldn't have done it without you.

I have only been able to write this book because of the therapists and coaches who have supported me since becoming a mother. Too many to mention, but a special thank you to Gurmukh Khalsa, Alister Gray, Karen Ramsay-Smith, Donna Lancaster, Laura Pringle, Lucy P, and Sheryl Close for being my emotional support team. I hope I've done you proud and walked the walk. Thank you to my gorgeous breathwork teacher and friend Ellie Taylor – I had many visions of this book in your classes.

Until I sat down to write, I had no idea of how vulnerable it feels to put your thoughts and stories onto a page. Thank you, Amy Warren, for being the book coach of dreams and holding my hand through those early 'Can I really do this?' wobbles. Amy, your input, expertise, friendship, and kindness has been invaluable – thank you. Thank you to Amy Meekings for being the first friend I sent the full manuscript to – thank you for your time, insightful feedback and support, it means the world. Thank you to my best friend Anna Kilmurray – a friendship like ours doesn't happen very often. Thank you for laughing with me (and at me), supporting me, and loving me unconditionally. Thank you to all my gorgeous friends new and old for your endless encouragement, support, last-minute playdates when I was on a deadline, and funny replies to my 'Can I really do this?' WhatsApps. Special thanks to Emma Worrollo, Emily Carr, Gina Felce, and Jo Sperryn for your support, guidance, and our monthly support sessions. I couldn't have done it without you.

To my agents at Bev James Management, Bev, Tom, and Liz. I still can't quite believe you took me on among your star-studded roster and I'm so endlessly grateful you did. Tom, thank you for always being the voice of reason with my 'creative' ideas and continually lifting me out of many wobbles.

Thank you to the whole team at HQ, especially Lisa, Emma, Danielle, Dawn, Komal, and Emily. Your passion for this book has been so incredible; thank you for the hard work and perseverance it's taken to get this book out there. Thank you to Ros Dundas for being the best PR there is.

To my family – Mum and Dad, thank you for always being there. Mum, thank you for letting me share a few of our stories with the world. You are ever an inspiration to me of what is possible with courage. Thank you for all your support and help with the girls. Dad, you often said to me, 'Someone has to have their dream job, why not you?' Well, I did it; thank you for planting that seed in me so young. To my brother, Andrew, thank you for your support. To my in-laws, Clare and Ian, thank you for your kindness and support (and for having the girls stay with you for a whole week when my deadline was looming!). I appreciate you.

Finally, thank you to my world – Guy, Jessie and Rose. To my husband, Guy – thank you for your unconditional support, for believing in me, guiding me, and loving me. I love you. Thank you for being my inspiration of what is possible when you believe in yourself. Thank you for being the first person to read my words and reading every single sentence since. Thank you for all the meals cooked, pick-ups done, and park trips taken so I could get this book written. I promise I won't do the next one in the summer holidays! To Jessie and Rose – words can't express how much I love you. Thank you for choosing me to be your mother. Thank you for helping me become the woman I was always meant to be. Thank you for being yourselves. I can't believe I get to watch you grow into the women you're meant to be. What a privilege. I hope one day you read this book and know that it was all because of you.

Further learning and resources

The Motherkind *podcast*

There are over 450 episodes covering everything in this book, and more. I release two new episodes a week, so make sure you subscribe so you never miss an episode.

Listen on: Spotify, Apple, Amazon Music, or wherever you get your podcasts.

On matrescence

Amy Taylor-Kabbaz, *Mama Rising: Discovering the New You Through Motherhood*, Hay House, 2019

Chelsea Conaboy, *Mother Brain: How Neuroscience Is Rewriting the Story of Parenthood*, Henry Holt & Co., 2022

Lucy Jones, *Matrescence: On the Metamorphosis of Pregnancy, Childbirth and Motherhood*, Allen Lane, 2023

Dr Oscar Serrallach, *The Postnatal Depletion Cure: A Complete Guide to Rebuilding Your Health and Reclaiming Your Energy for Mothers of Newborns, Toddlers and Young Children*, Grand Central Life & Style, 2018

On motherhood in society

Eliane Glaser, *Motherhood: A Manifesto*, Fourth Estate, 2021

Eve Rodsky, *Fair Play: A Game-Changing Solution for When You Have Too Much to Do (and More Life to Live)*, Quercus, 2019

Joeli Brearley, *The Motherhood Penalty: How to Stop Motherhood Being the Kiss of Death for Your Career*, Simon & Schuster UK, 2022

Dr Pragya Agarwal, *(M)otherhood: On the Choices of Being a Woman*, Canongate, 2021

Reshma Saujani, *Pay Up: The Future of Women and Work (and Why It's Different Than You Think)*, Atria/One Signal Publishers, 2022

On self-belief and compassion

Bruce Lipton, *The Biology of Belief: Unleashing the Power of Consciousness, Matter & Miracles*, Cygnus Books, 2005

Jen Sincero, *You Are a Badass: How to Stop Doubting Your Greatness and Start Living an Awesome Life*, Running Press, 2013

Dr Kristin Neff, *Self-Compassion: Stop Beating Yourself Up and Leave Insecurity Behind*, Hodder & Stoughton, 2011

Lisa Olivera, *Already Enough: A Path to Self-Acceptance*, Profile Books, 2022

Mel Robbins, *The High 5 Habit: Take Control of Your Life with One Simple Habit*, Hay House UK, 2021

Shahroo Izadi, *The Kindness Method: Changing Habits for Good*, Bluebird, 2018

On boundaries, perfectionism, and people pleasing

Brené Brown, *The Gifts of Imperfection: Let Go of Who You Think You're Supposed to Be and Embrace Who You Are*, Hazelden Publishing, 2010

Emma Reed Turrell, *Please Yourself: How to Stop People-Pleasing & Transform the Way You Live*, Fourth Estate, 2021

Kate Northrup, *Do Less: A Revolutionary Approach to Time and Energy Management for Busy Moms*, Hay House, 2019

Melissa Urban, *The Book of Boundaries: Set the Limits That Will Set You Free*, Vermilion, 2022

Tamu Thomas, *Women Who Work Too Much: Break Free from Toxic Productivity and Find Your Joy*, Hay House, 2024

On developing emotional skills

Anna Mathur, *Raising a Happier Mother: How to Find Balance, Feel Good and See Your Children Flourish as a Result*, Penguin Life, 2023

Dr Emma Svanberg, *Parenting for Humans: How to Parent the Child You Have, As the Person You Are*, Vermilion, 2023

Dr Julie Smith, *Why Has Nobody Told Me This Before?: Everyday Tools for Life's Ups and Downs*, Michael Joseph, 2022

Peter Levine, *Waking the Tiger: Healing Trauma*, North Atlantic Books, 1997

Philippa Perry, *The Book You Wish Your Parents Had Read (and Your Children Will Be Glad That You Did)*, Penguin Life, 2019

Dr Soph Mort, *A Manual for Being Human: What Makes Us Who We Are, Why it Matters and Practical Advice for a Happier Life*, Gallery Books, 2021

On values

Mark Manson, *The Subtle Art of Not Giving a F*ck: A Counterintuitive Approach to Living a Good Life*, Harper, 2016

Michelle Obama, *The Light We Carry: Overcoming in Uncertain Times*, Viking, 2022

Susan Jeffers, *Feel the Fear and Do it Anyway: Dynamic Techniques for Turning Fear, Indecision, and Anger into Power, Action and Love*, Thomson Learning, 1987

On energy and wellness

Dr Caroline Boyd, *Mindful New Mum: A Mind-Body Approach to the Highs and Lows of Motherhood*, DK, 2022

Emily and Amelia Nagoski, *Burnout: The Secret to Solving the Stress Cycle*, Vermilion, 2019

Dr Rangan Chatterjee, *Feel Better in 5: Your Daily Plan to Feel Great for Life*, Penguin Life, 2019

Suzy Reading, *The Self-Care Revolution: Smart Habits & Simple Practices to Allow You to Flourish*, Aster, 2017

On breaking generational cycles

Dr Becky, *Good Inside: A Guide to Becoming the Parent You Want to Be*, Harper, 2022

Donna Lancaster, *Wise Words for Women*, Ebury Press, 2023

Glennon Doyle, *Untamed: Stop Pleasing, Start Living*, Vermilion, 2020

Julia Samuel, *Every Family Has a Story: How We Inherit Love and Loss*, Penguin Life, 2022

Mark Wolynn, *It Didn't Start with You: How Inherited Family Trauma Shapes Who We Are and How to End the Cycle*, Viking, 2016

Dr Nicole LePera, *How to Do the Work: Recognize Your Patterns, Heal from Your Past, and Create Your Self*, Harper Wave, 2021

Dr Shefali, *The Conscious Parent: Transforming Ourselves, Empowering Our Children*, Yellow Kite, 2015

References

1. Invisible Mothers. (2023). https://invisible-mothers.peanut-app.io/
2. Rowland, K. (2018). We Are Multitudes. Aeon. https://aeon.co/essays/microchimerism-how-pregnancy-changes-the-mothers-very-dna
3. Hoekzema, E., Barba-Müller, E., Pozzobon, C. et al. (2016). Pregnancy leads to long-lasting changes in human brain structure. *Nature Neuroscience,* vol. 20, 287–296. https://doi.org/10.1038/nn.4458
4. Kim P. (2016). Human Maternal Brain Plasticity: Adaptation to Parenting. *Directions for Child and Adolescent Development,* vol. 153, 47–58. https://doi.org/10.1002/cad.20168
5. Caruso, C. (2016). Pregnancy Causes Lasting Changes in a Woman's Brain. *Scientific American.* https://www.scientificamerican.com/article/pregnancy-causes-lasting-changes-in-a-womans-brain/
6. Raspovic, A.M., Prichard, I., Yager, Z., & Hart, L.M. (2020). Mothers' experiences of the relationship between body image and exercise, 0–5 years postpartum: A qualitative study. *Body Image,* vol. 35, 41–52. https://doi.org/10.1016/j.bodyim.2020.08.003
7. Invisible Mothers. (2023). https://invisible-mothers.peanut-app.io/
8. Morse, G. (2002). Hidden Minds. *Harvard Business Review.* https://hbr.org/2002/06/hiddenminds#:~:text=Probably%2095%25%20of%20all%20cognition,visible%20and%20easy%20to%20access

9. Zaltman, G. (2003). How Customers Think: Essential Insights into the Mind of the Market. *Audio-Tech Business Book Summaries,* vol. 12. http://magnatar.nl/Magnatar/Brain_food/Artikelen/2011/8/18_ Marketing_Metaphoria_-_Zaltman_files/howcustomersthink.pdf

10. Everett, S. (2021). The Brainwave Frequencies Which Underlie Language Development. Elite Learning. https://www.elitelearning. com/resource-center/rehabilitation-therapy/occupational-therapy/ the-brainwave-frequencies-which-underlie-language-development/

11. The Joy Project. https://www.ulta.com/discover/beauty-reads/ joy-project/joy-study

12. Motherly's 2021 State of Motherhood Survey Results (2021). https://www.mother.ly/news/2021-state-of-motherhood-survey/

13. Maftei, A., Lăzărescu, G. (2022). Times Are Harsh, Be Kind to Yourself! Anxiety, Life Satisfaction, and the Mediating Role of Self-Compassion. *Frontiers in Psychology,* vol. 13. https://doi. org/10.3389/fpsyg.2022.915524

14. Comaford, C. (2012). Got Inner Peace? 5 Ways to Get it Now. *Forbes.* https://www.forbes.com/sites/ christinecomaford/2012/04/04/got-inner-peace-5-ways-to-get-it-now/?sh=767455bf6672

15. Fairbrother, N., Martin, R., & Challacombe, F. (2022). Unwanted, Intrusive Thoughts of Infant-Related Harm. *Key Topics in Perinatal Mental Health,* 93–112.

16. Motherly's 2021 State of Motherhood Survey Results (2021). https://www.mother.ly/news/2021-state-of-motherhood-survey/

17. Invisible Mothers. (2023). https://invisible-mothers.peanut-app.io/

18. Ennis, L. R. (Ed.). (2014). *Intensive Mothering: The Cultural Contradictions of Modern Motherhood.* Demeter Press. https:// www.jstor.org/stable/j.ctt1rrd8rb

19. Bauer, L., Wang, S. (2023). Prime-Age Women Are Going Above and Beyond in the Labor Market Recovery. The Hamilton Project. https://www.hamiltonproject.org/publication/post/

prime-age-women-are-going-above-and-beyond-in-the-labor-
market-recovery/

20. Miller, C. (2018). The Relentlessness of Modern Parenting. *New York Times*. https://www.nytimes.com/2018/12/25/upshot/the-relentlessness-of-modern-parenting.html

21. Walthery, P., Chung, H. (2021). Sharing of childcare and wellbeing outcomes: an empirical analysis. UK Cabinet Office.

22. Pressure to be a 'supermum' affecting women's mental health. Bupa. (2022). https://www.bupa.com/news/press-releases/2022/normal-mums#:~:text=New%20research%20from%20leading%20health,has%20affected%20their%20mental%20health.

23. Tucker, C.J., Finkelhor, D. (2015). The State of Interventions for Sibling Conflict and Aggression: A Systematic Review. *Trauma, Violence & Abuse I-II*. Sage. https://www.unh.edu/ccrc/sites/default/files/media/2022-02/trauma-violence-abuse-2015-tucker-1524838015622438.pdf

24. Cross, R., Dillon, K. (2023). The Hidden Toll of Microstress. *Harvard Business Review*. https://hbr.org/2023/02/the-hidden-toll-of-microstress

25. Nair, A. (2024). WhatsApp Statistics for 2024 – All You Need to Know. Verloop. https://verloop.io/blog/whatsapp-statistics-2024/#:~:text=A%20study%20showed%20that%2C%20on,per%20time%20of%20the%20day

26. Delahunty, S. (2020). Mummy Bloggers Perfect Parenting Tropes Driving Mental Health Crisis. *PR Week*. https://www.prweek.com/article/1668274/mummy-bloggers-perfect-parenting-tropes-driving-mental-health-crisis

27. Instagram's user base grows to more than 500 million. (2016). Reuters https://www.reuters.com/article/us-facebook-instagram-users-idUSKCN0Z71LN

28. 7 Reasons to Break Your Smartphone Addiction. Piedmont. https://www.piedmont.org/living-real-change/

does-your-smartphone-cause-anxiety#:~:text=Why%20are%20
smartphones%20so%20addictive,and%20leads%20to%20a%20
letdown

29. Office for National Statistics. (2016, November 10). Women
    shoulder the responsibility of unpaid work. Retrieved from
    https://www.ons.gov.uk/employmentandlabourmarket/
    peopleinwork/earningsandworkinghours/articles/
    womenshouldertheresponsibilityofunpaidwork/2016-11-10

30. Invisible Mothers. (2023). https://invisible-mothers.peanut-app.io/

31. Carmo, C., Oliveira, D., Brás, M., & Faísca, L. (2021). The
    Influence of Parental Perfectionism and Parenting Styles on Child
    Perfectionism. *Children*, vol. 8 (9), 777. https://doi.org/10.3390/
    children8090777

32. Delahunty, S. (2020). Mummy Bloggers Perfect Parenting Tropes
    Driving Mental Health Crisis. *PR Week*. https://www.prweek.
    com/article/1668274/mummy-bloggers-perfect-parenting-tropes-
    driving-mental-health-crisis

33. Johnson, P. (2021). Good Enough Parenting. *Forest for the Trees
    Perinatal Psychology*. https://forestpsychology.com.au/good-
    enough-parenting

34. Sizensky, V. (2015*). New Survey: Moms Are Putting Their Health
    Last. healthywomen. https://www.healthywomen.org/content/
    article/new-survey-moms-are-putting-their-health-last

35. Peanut Gives Voice to Motherhood in New 'Invisible Mothers'
    Campaign. (2023). Little Black Book. https://lbbonline.com/news/
    peanut-gives-voice-to-motherhood-in-new-invisible-mothers-
    campaign/

36. Mallick, M. (2021). Moms are living in an extraordinary era of
    burnout. Motherly. https://www.mother.ly/parenting/moms-
    suffering-from-pandemic-burnout/

37. Trend of Increased Alcohol Consumption Held Steady as
    Pandemic Dragged On, New Survey Results Show. (2021). PR

Newswire. https://www.prnewswire.com/news-releases/trend-
of-increased-alcohol-consumption-held-steady-as-pandemic-
dragged-on-new-survey-results-show-301353729.html

38. Managing Adult Sleep With Baby on Board. Brevard Health. https://
    brevardhealth.org/blog/managing-adult-sleep-with-baby-on-board/

39. Kitamura, S., Katayose, Y., Nakazaki, K., Motomura, Y., Oba, K.,
    Katsunuma, R., Terasawa, Y., Enomoto, M., Moriguchi, Y., Hida,
    A., & Mishima, K. (2016). Estimating individual optimal sleep
    duration and potential sleep debt. *Scientific Reports*, vol. 6, 35812.
    https://doi.org/10.1038/srep35812

40. Still feeling good: The US wellness market continues to boom.
    (2022). McKinsey & Company. https://www.mckinsey.com/
    industries/consumer-packaged-goods/our-insights/still-feeling-
    good-the-us-wellness-market-continues-to-boom

41. Petter, O. (2018). Being a mother is equivalent to 2.5 full-time
    jobs, survey finds. *Independent*. https://www.independent.co.uk/
    life-style/health-and-families/mother-equivalent-2-jobs-full-time-
    childcare-98-hours-work-mum-survey-a8258676.html

42. Patel, J., Patel, P. (2019). Consequences of Repression of Emotion:
    Physical Health, Mental Health and General Well Being.
    International Journal of Psychotherapy Practice and Research, vol.
    1 (3), 16–21. https://doi.org/10.14302/issn.2574-612X.ijpr-18-2564

43. Patel, J., Patel, P. (2019). Consequences of Repression of Emotion:
    Physical Health, Mental Health and General Well Being.
    International Journal of Psychotherapy Practice and Research, vol.
    1 (3), 16-21. https://doi.org/10.14302/issn.2574-612X.ijpr-18-2564

44. Ganguly, R. (2023). How to Supercharge Your Life With
    Gratitude. Axelerant. https://www.axelerant.com/blog/
    gratitude-practice#:~:text=Research%20shows%20practicing%20
    gratitude%20can,35%25%20reduction%20in%20depressive%20
    symptoms.

45. Mom guilt: 94 percent of us have it. Can we ditch it for a week?

(2011). Today.com. https://www.today.com/parents/mom-guilt-94-percent-us-have-it-can-we-ditch-1c7399369

46. Mom guilt: 94 percent of us have it. Can we ditch it for a week? (2011). Today.com. https://www.today.com/parents/mom-guilt-94-percent-us-have-it-can-we-ditch-1c7399369

47. Working mothers feel higher levels of guilt due to internalised gender stereotypes compared to fathers, reveals new study. (2022). British Psychological Society. https://www.bps.org.uk/news/working-mothers-feel-higher-levels-guilt-due-internalised-gender-stereotypes-compared-fathers

48. Brearley, J. Mothers Are Overdue a Revolution of Their Own. In: Gillard, J. et al. (2023). *Essays on Equality: The politics of childcare.* The Global Institute for Women's Leadership. https://www.kcl.ac.uk/news/mothers-are-overdue-a-revolution-of-their-own

49. Hess, A. J. (2017). Here's Why Lottery Winners Go Broke. CNBC. https://www.cnbc.com/2017/08/25/heres-why-lottery-winners-go-broke.html

50. Research reveals how many decisions you make in a day and which ones are the most difficult. (2022). *Metro.* https://metro.co.uk/2022/08/09/study-reveals-how-many-decisions-we-make-each-day-17150428/#:~:text=It%20turns%20out%20that%20we,what%20to%20wear%20and%20watch

51. Hamilton, D. (2020). The Most Contagious Thing Is Kindness. https://drdavidhamilton.com/the-most-contagious-thing-is-kindness/#:~:text=That%27s%205%20x%205%20x,They%27re%20are

52. Bradt, S. (2021). Wandering Mind Not a Happy Mind. *Harvard Gazette.* https://news.harvard.edu/gazette/story/2010/11/wandering-mind-not-a-happy-mind/

53. Bradt, S. (2021). Wandering Mind not a Happy Mind. *Harvard Gazette.* https://news.harvard.edu/gazette/story/2010/11/wandering-mind-not-a-happy-mind/

Index